THINK LIKE AN HERBALIST

A Practical Guide to Healing Common Health Problems and Resolving the Ones You Already Have

by

Amelia South

Certified Herbalist and Gut Health Restoration Specialist

Edited by Arecales Wind

Cover Artwork and Design by Gail Nelson

South, Amelia Think Like an Herbalist

Second edition

amelia@nobsherbalist.com

Published in the United States of America by Black Sun Publishing

Black Sun Publishing

Danielson, CT 06239

ISBN-13: 979-8-9944322-0-4

Special thanks to

Julian Christian M.S., L.A., C.M.T.

Elizabeth P. Russell, Herbalist

Bryan Redfield

Layne Whitley (who came up with the title)

Also, to Sajah Popham and Paul Bergner, two of my favorite herbal teachers (who probably have no idea who I am).

Table of Contents

Disclaimer

The content presented in this book is for informational purposes only and is not intended to serve as medical advice or a substitute for professional medical consultation. I am not a licensed medical doctor or a clinical herbalist (at this time). The information contained herein is a blend of folk wisdom, general health knowledge, and personal experiences related to herbal remedies and health management.

Please be aware that individual responses to herbs and remedies can vary significantly. What may be beneficial to one person may not be effective or could potentially cause an adverse reaction in another. Allergic reactions and other sensitivities to herbs and remedies are possible. Therefore, it is crucial to exercise caution when introducing new herbs or remedies into your regimen. It is recommended to start with a small dose, increasing incrementally, to gauge your body's response.

By purchasing or using this book, you acknowledge and agree that neither Amelia South nor Black Sun Farm shall be held liable for any adverse effects, injuries, or medical issues that may arise from the application of the information provided. Always consult with a qualified healthcare professional before making any change to your health or wellness routine.

This disclaimer is intended to protect both the author and publisher and to ensure that readers make informed decisions regarding their health and well-being.

Introduction

This book is everything I wish I had known by the time I was 20.

When we hit our 40s, so many of us think, "Oh, if only I knew this sooner in life!" It takes 20+ years to gain the experiential knowledge you attain through trial and error. But can you imagine if someone had written it all down once they figured it out, traveled back in time, and handed it to you? You know, the simple daily stuff that you could have used to help you make informed decisions about your health for the rest of your life.

I imagine myself standing outside the club I used to go to, wearing fishnets, chunky black heels, and a skirt that barely covered my ass. It's 10 p.m., and I'm waiting to go inside when some older lady who looks like a slightly fatter and older version of me runs out of the alleyway, shoves this book into my coat pocket, and in a voice that brooks no argument says, "Read this when you get home, and don't lose it!" I stare at her, bewildered, and blink a few times as she kisses me on the forehead, turns around, and disappears back into the night.

If that had actually happened and I had read this very book back then (after getting home from dancing, of course), I would not have made half the mistakes I have made over the last 20 years. I went through years' worth of trial, error, study, and experience so I can feel confident now showing you how to avoid the same mistakes I made.

After years of assisting clients, customers, and people on social media, I've observed that many people lack certain wisdom about their own health. Because I have seen such a large gap in human knowledge, and because I'm a farmer, herbalist, and one of those strange people who collects a thousand facts in their head until it's just the right time to let one loose, I'm writing this all down for you. From me: an actual human with actual human knowledge.

What you're getting here is a combination of street smarts and book knowledge. I'm helping you reverse engineer your problems in order to solve them, not just suggesting herbs that will mask the symptoms you are experiencing. While I absolutely love to work with herbs (and will tell you my favorite ones to work with), my methods encourage you to focus the majority of your effort on healing the internal imbalances in your body. By taking this approach, your symptoms begin to diminish, making it so that you don't need to rely solely on herbs to manage your health.

This book is organized into two parts:

Part One discusses the prevention of problems and diseases—what you can do, no matter how healthy you are (or are not) right now, to help improve your health in general.

Part Two offers my solutions to some of the most common ailments people face today. The topics covered in Part Two are primarily based on the long list of complaints people have come to me with over the past few years as well as my own personal health experiences.

Important Note: as of this writing, I practice Western Herbalism. I don't discuss Traditional Chinese Medicine or Ayurveda in this book.

I do NOT know everything. I'm an herbalist, not a doctor. However, I HAVE studied a vast range of subjects and am educated in many different areas. I will not tell you anything unless it's something I've done, I've experienced myself, or it's backed by research. I will cite my sources, so you are able to do your own research, which I encourage you to do. Sometimes, the source of my information is something I learned the hard way, by going through it myself. I spent the last 11+ years working on organic farms and inside greenhouse operations, all while raising two children through divorce, a new relationship, and divorce again.

Your mental and emotional health are critical to your physical health. This isn't something anyone tells you right out of the gate, unless you've already spent most of your childhood in therapy. My hot take on therapy: If you've been seeing the same therapist for three years or more and you're still not seeing improvement or feeling better, you need a different therapist. In such an instance, it should be obvious that that particular person cannot help you. Save yourself the energy, time, and money—find someone who *can*.

In this book, I do not use a lot of flowery language or descriptions. Books that are written in that style are lovely, but I aim to accomplish something different here. I'm writing this 1) to give you practical advice you can look up as quickly as possible and 2) to give you the best starting point before you delve more deeply into researching your specific problem with the guidance of more in-depth resources.

That's the big thing I'm giving you here: my resources. I've been doing this long enough to know who to trust as a reliable source of information. I know which books were written by real humans (not AI) who have more extensive and specialized knowledge than you may find in this book. Knowing which authors and books are relevant to you, you can acquire them and build your own library the same way I have.

If I don't know the answer to something, where would I look up more information on that subject? How would I go about finding the answers? Which sources do I trust? Here, I tell you the resources (books, websites, etc.) I would utilize when doing research on the various topics we cover. Fear not! These aren't hidden resources that you can only access with a special key to the Library of Congress. In fact, a number of the resources I share are free to access online.

Of course, you are more than welcome to find alternative resources if mine do not suit you. You can even send me an email about books, websites, resources, or research you know of that you think I should know about. I'm open to continual learning; I hope you are too.

I want this book to be your head start to learning how to heal yourself and others based on how I have done it for myself. At some point while reading this book, I hope you say, "Holy crap, I never thought of that!" Let the information herein flip on a light bulb in your brain—one that lets you know you have the ability to heal yourself, if only you employ the correct methods. If you are a parent, read this book, and then give it to your child when they're preparing to venture out into the world on their own.

Note: This book does not contain all the same information as my Gut Healing Protocol. While you can glean a lot of what you need to know about healing your gut from this book, it **does not** replace my Gut Healing Protocol, in which I go into more depth and specifics about healing your gut.

If all you plan to do is skip around in this book to the parts you think are relevant to you, read the names of a few herbs, begin taking them, and all your health problems will be cured, then you will be sorely disappointed. Taking such an approach will not only waste your time but will also have wasted your money in purchasing this book.

If you live in the United States, you're most likely familiar with a system of healthcare known as allopathic medicine (or conventional medicine). With this approach, you wait until you begin experiencing a problem or symptom; then, you search for a solution to your problem or symptom via drugs, herbs, surgery, therapy, etc.

I personally take a holistic approach to solving my problems and when helping others. Rather than only focusing on the problem or symptom, I look at the WHOLE person. I ask you all kinds of questions when we chat in our consultation, such as, "What's your diet like? How often do you exercise? Are you in a happy relationship? How was your childhood? How often do you poop?" Along with any other questions that will help give me a picture of who you are and where you're coming from health-wise.

I wrote this book to show you what you need to do to heal your entire body, not just the condition or symptoms you're most concerned with at the moment. I do my best to focus on resolving the root cause of each problem I encounter. Part Two of this book is organized by ailments, organs, and body systems, with each section serving as a quick guide and offering you a place to start in your research.

From there, you can refer to the References, Indispensable Reading, Additional Resources, and Recommended Products sections at the end of the book, where you can find information on all citations and hyperlinks included throughout the text. The end of the book also contains a section with Links and QR Codes you can scan with your smart phone (in the physical copy of this book) to products I personally use and recommend as well as educational videos and more.

I'm not a scientist writing a dissertation; I'm a regular woman who knows a lot of things that can help you start healing your physical and mental problems naturally, without having to spend three weeks combing through a mountain of resources. As the title states, I'm here to help you start *thinking* like an herbalist.

Warnings:

I'm writing both facts and my opinions in this book, most of which are based on scientific research. Throughout the text and in my references page, I have cited my resources so they are easily accessible to you, dear reader, for further inspection, investigation, and research.

I am not a vegan or vegetarian. I believe eating meat is a healthy part of the human diet when done ethically. I do not judge you if you are a vegan or vegetarian; just be aware that this book is not catered to the vegan or vegetarian diet. I'm an omnivore, so I'm writing from that perspective.

If you're reading this book, I'm assuming you are a resident of the United States or Canada. I practice Western Herbalism, and I (mostly) use Americanized spelling. Where I live, it is correct to say "an herbalist" rather than "a herbalist," even though I know the latter is correct in other countries.

The etymology of pronouncing the "h" at the beginning of certain words and not others is interesting. It has to do with the fact that England was conquered by the French nearly 1000 years ago, and over the years, adopted many French phrases and pronunciations into the English language.

Whether you're from North America or somewhere else across the globe, I greatly appreciate your reading my book.

Most importantly, I wrote this book to help people, not to harm anyone or pretend I'm a doctor. I hope my book accomplishes this in an accessible, comprehensible, and enjoyable way!

Now, on to the fun part…

Part One: Prevention

The Foundation of Your Health

I'm an herbalist. Lots of people treat me the same way they would treat a doctor, asking me questions about how to heal this ailment, that organ system, or a weird rash they have on their thigh. Few of them care about anything but the answer they want to hear, which is some version of "Just take this plant extract for two weeks and you'll be cured!" That's not what I'm going to tell you.

I have gone through MANY of the same problems that I've outlined inside this book, so when I offer you a personal anecdote or suggestion on how to heal whatever problem we're addressing, know that it's usually first-hand, experiential knowledge based on treating myself, my family, and many clients. I do, of course, adhere to the expertise of the many herbal teachers I have studied with as well. And whenever fitting, I will point you toward their material to learn more.

I help as many people as I can, to the best of my ability, because I *want* to help. I want people to find relief in natural remedies. I want to renew their faith in the healing power of plants. Unfortunately, it's not just "herbal remedies" that they need. And that's where my suggestions meet resistance.

"What do you mean I need to stop eating Hot Pockets? That's my favorite food!" "But I can't give up soda. Besides, it says 'zero sugar' on the package. Isn't that good enough?" "I simply *can't* stop eating string cheese; I don't care what you say."

These are just a few of the objections I have been met with from people who have asked me for health advice on how to cure one issue or another. Often, they don't want to make the changes that need to be made to see improvements in their specific condition and general health.

I will continue to shout this from the rooftops as long as I live: FOOD IS MEDICINE.

We've all heard the phrase "You are what you eat." In reality, you are what your body **absorbs**—whether that's through your digestive tract (food and drink), your skin (cosmetics, lotions, and sprays), or your mucous membranes (tinctures and homeopathic tablets).

Think of your body like a house: Your stomach/digestive tract is the foundation your house (and health) needs to stand upon. Herbs and herbal remedies are like the siding on your house. The siding serves as a support, making your house strong and secure, but you'd technically survive without it.

The siding isn't going to do you much good without a strong, solid house and foundation to sit upon. The same goes for herbal remedies. Herbs can help manage your symptoms, support your internal systems, and even add some nutrition to your diet. However, taking a bunch of herbs without eating a healthy diet and making sure you have a fully functioning microbiome is like if you tried to put out a bonfire with a box of baking soda. The approach, although helpful in less extreme circumstances, is totally ineffective given the sheer magnitude of the problem.

To achieve good health and the best quality of life you can have, you must attend to the foundation of your health: your digestive tract and gut microbiome. Without addressing these areas of your health first and foremost, you are overlooking a system that affects virtually every other system in your body.

To simplify, gut balance facilitates good health, while gut dysbiosis spells trouble in the form of ailments, imbalances, inflammation, and chronic health issues.

Chapter 1: A Little Background on How Your Body Works

Your body needs vitamins and minerals to function properly. Without the right balance of vitamins and minerals, you begin to experience an array of problems. Something as simple as a vitamin deficiency could be the root cause behind your symptoms, and you wouldn't even realize it until someone like me brings it to your attention.

Did you know that your body requires vitamins A and K to absorb the vitamin D it gets? And that your body cannot absorb vitamins A and K without enough vitamin D available? Or that you need enough calcium in your body to absorb magnesium, and vice versa? Correcting vitamin deficiency might sound like something a nutritionist is trying to shove down your throat (pun intended), but it's nothing to take lightly.

This is the most important thing for you to remember: NO herb or combination of herbs can fix or replace a nutritional deficiency. There are herbs that can help, but it's the right combination of diet and exercise that can heal you.

When I was in college and for the few years after that when I was out in the world "on my own," I ate whatever I wanted, whenever I wanted, slept whenever I wanted, and went wherever I wanted (that I could afford to go). And like many young people do during that stage of life, I drank alcohol profusely when I was around friends. I was living the life!

I *also* had chronic yeast infections and irregular bowel movements. In 2006, I ended up with HPV after only five sexual partners. You see, HPV is passed to women from men. Often, men don't show any signs or symptoms, so they don't know they have it. Women, however, end up with the possibility of developing genital warts (which I, thankfully, never had) and a much higher chance of developing cervical cancer. I did develop abnormal cells on my cervix and underwent LEEP surgery to have the section removed.

LEEP surgery is wildly underplayed by most gynecologists as a run-of-the-mill procedure, but if the doctor doesn't do it *exactly* right, the surgery can result in pain, bleeding, and an inability to experience sexual pleasure or orgasm for the rest of the woman's life. I thank the universe every day that I did not suffer these issues from having the surgery done. I am part of a LEEP support group online, though, as I have had some lasting effects from the procedure. I hear horror stories of women whose doctors do not listen to them or do not believe their side-effect symptoms. Losing sexual function is no joke!

Despite the adverse effects, I continued eating whatever I wanted and just accepted that I would have a chronic yeast problem for the rest of my life (even through my first pregnancy). That was my life until I watched a documentary called *Fat Head* in 2011. It changed my perceptions regarding my diet entirely. From that point on, I made the most important decision of my life: I got into self-help.

It did not matter to me that my loved ones thought it was goofy or did not care to join me. It did not matter to me what anyone thought because I was working on myself for myself. By the time I reached age 38, I had an epiphany that brought me out of **victim mode** once and for all. Through what I can only safely describe as a mental breakdown, I was forced to realize, understand, and accept that if I took responsibility for myself and my actions, then no one could control me anymore. [Note: I just wrote an entire book about this experience!]

Once I began to see that my food choices and alcohol consumption were what was causing my health problems, I no longer had the attitude that things were "happening *to* me." I was able to take my power back. No longer did I say, "The booze made me sick." I now said, "My decision to drink booze led me to become sick." No longer did I say that someone manipulated me emotionally and financially. I now said, "I allowed someone to manipulate me." Framing things in this way allowed me to take back control of my life.

I want you to be able to do this too. I want you to see that your decisions about what you do with your body are a huge contributor to your health problems (both mental and physical). The good news is that means YOU have the power to change your decisions and, by extension, your entire life.

If someone asks me, "What herb can I take for my depression so I don't have to take drugs?" My answer is, "How much sunlight are you getting? Do you have enough vitamin D in your body? Do you ever go outside in the forest and just take a walk? What quality of sleep are you typically getting? What's your diet like?"

The majority of people don't want to hear these questions. They want me to say, "Oh, take some ashwagandha for a few weeks, and you'll be healed!" But I'm not going to lie to you to sell you herbs that you don't need. The other problem most healers gloss over is one of the most important of all: You can try all the diet and exercise changes you want, **but until you change your mindset**, all other changes will only yield temporary relief.

How do you change your mindset? Well, the first step is to accept that you need help. People who get into self-help to any extent will typically see more success than those who want a quick fix to their problems. Once you realize, understand, and accept that seeking out help from a qualified person or resource is what you need, everything changes. You stop being the victim and start taking back control of your life and your reality.

Once you find help and know what you need to do, you also have to decide to go through with it. I have sold hundreds of copies of my Gut Healing Protocol, and in it, on the very last page, is my version of an "easy button" to show the client how to move past whatever is blocking them from wanting to go through with making the suggested changes.

Few people take advantage of it. They ignore it as part of the program, dismissing it as some woo-woo concept that doesn't matter because it's not a food- or supplement-based suggestion. But if you truly know that your subconscious thoughts control everything you do, you'll take my "easy button" to heart and try it for yourself.

Every human body is different. I don't know your body, what you look like, what your diet is like, your lifestyle, your medical history, what medications you're taking, what your body's constitution is, or any of the other information I would need to assess the problems you're experiencing. When I give someone a consultation, after assessing their needs, I give them their own personalized "easy button" to help them change their subconscious programming and become the person they were truly meant to be in body, mind, and soul.

One final note: If you are currently taking any pharmaceutical medication, it's critical that you research any potential herb-drug interactions that could potentially occur. The herbal remedies I talk about in this book are written for someone who is **not** on any medication. **It's your responsibility to research the safety of taking any herbal remedies for your specific body and situation.** I offer many additional resources at the end of the book that can assist you in your research.

This book does **NOT** replace a consultation with a qualified herbalist, naturopath, or doctor. It is meant to be utilized as a reference to help you achieve relief while you're waiting to have an appointment with someone who can help you specifically.

If you're in generally good health and want to make sure you stay that way, the information in this book may provide you with the missing pieces you need to maintain balance and harmony inside your body for the foreseeable future.

I don't want any of you, my readers, to think that buying my book means you'll never need to go to the doctor or seek health advice from anyone ever again. At the same time, I stand behind my research and experience, expecting that you will find value in the coming pages.

Chapter 2: Do You Need a Doctor?

I want to make this very clear: Sometimes, you DO need a doctor.

If you're out in a field and accidentally step on an old chunk of steel left there in the 60s when Uncle Jimbo tore the tractor apart and left parts all over the place, you're going to want a doctor to sew your toe back on and give you a tetanus shot.

If you have a sharp pain in your leg every time you move it, and it sends waves of nausea through your body to the point you can hardly breathe or move, you want to have a doctor run some tests to figure out why.

If you (like me) feel a lump in your throat that hurts when you swallow and gets worse over time, you want to see a doctor and ask for tests to find out why so you (also like me) can catch the *cancer* that may be growing there and have it removed before it has a chance to harm you.

DOCTORS are the ones who can order the TESTS you need to figure out what's making you feel sick or generally unwell. It's foolish to discount the usefulness of the entire medical industry and all the advances it's made over the last hundred years. The medical profession has its place. In some instances, they can save your life.

I don't want to be dependent on the pharmaceutical industry any more than you do. I completely agree that they are now one of the major ruling bodies in this world. The man who owns a drug company is basically a king. But we also need to accept that there are things we may not know that a doctor or hospital could potentially help us figure out.

I also know that many of the doctors and nurses who help people for a living are tired of their every move being scrutinized by the pharmaceutical industry and the for-profit hospital system. I'm writing down everything I've learned so that you can have a guide on ways to heal yourself and where to look for further information without needing a doctor at every sign of trouble.

I think we can both agree to respect doctors and nurses and all the knowledge they possess while also disliking and mistrusting the pharmaceutical industrial complex.

Now, on to the education!

There are two types of problems you may face: acute problems and chronic problems.

An **acute problem** is usually caused by an injury, virus, or accident. For example, you fell down while roller skating and threw your right shoulder out. It's super sore, your muscles and tendons are torn and painful to move, and you may have a minor hairline fracture that's not serious enough for a cast but does need some care. Or, you caught a bad virus on the airplane ride back from Italy, and now you haven't been able to shake this chesty, deep cough in your lungs, making your sides hurt and disrupting your sleep.

A **chronic problem** is something that either starts and never stops or builds up slowly over time. Maybe you twisted your knee a few years ago playing basketball, and it's been sore when you walk ever since. Maybe you used to be able to eat anything you wanted, but now you have diverticulitis, and if you're not careful, you get painful bowel flares that can last for weeks. Maybe you used to be just fine going to parties with your friends, but now even going for a walk down Main Street fills you with dread.

I freely admit that herbal remedies can help with many of the problems you may encounter over the course of your life. There are thousands of herbs out there, and I only work with a small portion of them. I am not about to tell you that pulling your hamstring back in 2019 caused your IBS. But I will tell you that you're going to get the most help from herbs and natural remedies if your gut is in good working order.

Take wild lettuce, for example. I make a badass wild lettuce tincture. Hundreds of my customers swear by it, but I have met people who say, "Yeah, it's okay, I guess." When I ask them why they think it doesn't work for them, almost every one of them tells me the same thing: "The wild lettuce isn't as strong as opiates."

NO KIDDING. Wild lettuce is a weed that grows in nature. Opium, while derived from a poppy plant, has been carefully processed into pharmaceutical-grade painkillers like fentanyl and OxyContin. It's highly addictive and stops pain better than just about anything. But it causes dependence and other complications, and it does *nothing* to address the root cause of your pain.

When I've been working out on the farm all day and I'm feeling tired and sore, I will come in after I'm finished and take some wild lettuce tincture, usually around dinner time. Because I eat a whole foods diet and do my utmost to make sure I have the right balance of nutrition in my body (I also don't drink, smoke, or do illicit drugs), the wild lettuce knocks my pain out *in seconds.* My lifestyle contributes more to my low levels of inflammation than any herb I take medicinally does.

Again, I know that may not be what you came here to hear. What you're here for is my list of remedies. But I have to explain all this to you before I offer you herbal remedies as a potential solution because I desperately need you to understand that herbs are not always the answer to your problems. Herbs are fantastic and are powerful healers! But sometimes herbs can cover up your problem the same way a drug will.

Here's another example: Your 3-year-old child is feeling unwell. You take his temperature, and he has a fever of 101.3°F. Do you go to the cupboard and get him some children's Tylenol? Or do you make him comfortable on the couch with a Disney movie and something to drink and allow the fever to run its course?

Hopefully you choose the second option. Giving a child Tylenol or ibuprofen for a fever under 101.3°F is just going to mask the symptoms of whatever virus or bacteria his body is trying to fight off. The drug ends up making the child feel better for a while, stopping the body from fighting off the infection (which is what the fever does). It ends up making their sickness last days and days longer, or possibly weeks, rather than being over when the fever kills off the pathogen.

(Note: This advice is for children over the age of one. For very young infants, in case of a bad fever, please consult your pediatrician.)

I will never tell you not to call a doctor if you think you or your child are sick beyond what you can handle at home. You should do whatever you feel is best for yourself, your child, or anyone else who is under your care. All I want to do is give you the confidence to occasionally say, "You know what? I think we'll be fine if we just take a day or two of rest and drink some herbal tea."

What I WILL say, after all this, is that there are some very common ailments that people regularly deal with that herb can help heal. And there are some simple remedies that I can offer you as a general go-to for these problems or symptoms. Herbs were mankind's first medicine, and I believe they will certainly be its last.

Chapter 3: Your Gut

Gut problems are no longer rare; in fact, they've become quite the epidemic. From constant bloating to brain fog, millions of people are living with symptoms they've been told are "normal." But they're not. Our modern lifestyles—packed with stress, sleep deprivation, and quick fixes from medications and antibiotics—have put our digestive systems under constant strain. Add to that the massive changes in our diet over the last few decades, and you have the perfect storm. So while food is more plentiful than ever, much of what we find at the grocery store is stripped of the nutrients our bodies, minds, and gut microbiomes need to truly function well.

A **microbiome** is the community of microorganisms (such as fungi, bacteria, and viruses) that exists in a particular environment. In humans, the term is often used to describe the microorganisms that live in or on a particular part of the body, such as the skin or gastrointestinal tract. Your gut microbiome is one of the most important parts of your body, as it affects your digestion, skin, weight, heart health, immune system, and brain function. In fact, because of all the microbes present in your gut, it is often referred to as your second brain!

The health of your gut microbiome is critical to the health of your entire body. The gut-skin connection is what tells me that your chronic dermatitis or eczema is related to a gut imbalance. The gut-brain connection is what tells me that your severe anxiety is due to an imbalance in your gut flora. Did you know that 90% of the serotonin produced in your body is created in your gut? Serotonin, the hormone that is partially responsible for regulating your digestion, mood, sleep, blood clotting, bone health, sexual desire, and wound healing, also depends on the health of your gut (Bektas et al., 2020).

Leaky gut (or increased intestinal permeability) is a HUGE problem for millions of people. Most people don't start experiencing the symptoms of leaky gut (which are numerous and varied) until their 30s, by which point such extensive damage has been done to their intestinal lining that it takes quite a bit of time and effort to repair.

Imagine your intestines are one of those long, skinny balloons, like the kind a clown makes balloon animals with. When the outside of the balloon (your intestines) is made of rubber, your digestive system is working properly and absorbing all the nutrition from your food. In other words, healthy intestines are impervious to permeation, acting as a barrier and not allowing bacteria or toxins to pass into your bloodstream (Bischoff et al., 2014).

If the outside of that balloon turns into something more akin to cheesecloth, little microscopic particles of food escape into other parts of your body. In response, your immune system says, "Oh crap! The ham sandwich you just ate is supposed to stay inside your digestive tract. It's not supposed to be out here touching all of your other organs." In response, your immune system attacks the escaped food particles to protect you. Over time, this leads to the development of one or multiple autoimmune conditions or other symptoms like IBS, eczema, rosacea, etc. (Sadowsky et al., 2023).

The most common causes of leaky gut are the overuse of antibiotics (commonly prescribed by doctors to treat the flu or a bacterial infection) and regularly drinking too much alcohol (having more than one alcoholic drink per week). In the second scenario, the alcohol travels through your stomach like a giant tsunami of death, killing a considerable amount of your gut's good bacteria. What you're left with is the strongest (and often the worst) bacteria having survived without any good bacteria to balance them out.

There are foods, teas, and supplements you can take that can help support your gut health, but the only lasting solution to leaky gut is a complete lifestyle overhaul. While lots of people eat yogurt or take acidophilus pills daily, relying on these alone is not nearly enough to reset and repair your digestive microbes. I recommend you take a high-quality, daily probiotic to help maintain a healthy gut microbiome, such as Silver Fern™ Ultimate Probiotic. Certain bacteria are essential for repopulating your gut, and this particular supplement supplies them well.

I outline the above changes and more, making them clear and easy, in my Gut Healing Protocol. I personally spent over ten years learning how to heal my gut problems, finding a solution when I finally tested out the right strain of probiotics that helped me heal my gut. I've since helped over 700 people heal their gut by following my Gut Healing Protocol.

As a way of saying thank you for buying my book, you can get my Gut Healing Protocol for 20% off by using the coupon code TLAHBOOK20 when you order it on my website (linked in the Additional Resources section at the end of the book).

Chapter 4: Nutrients—Vitamins and Minerals

Have you ever wondered how you can become deficient in key nutrients even when your diet predominately consists of whole foods and you're taking a daily vitamin? Well, there's more to nutrition than just putting the right stuff into your body. The importance of getting the right vitamins and minerals through whole food sources can be traced back to something called **bioavailability**. When something is bioavailable, it means the present nutrients are in a form that your body can actually absorb.

For instance, if you find you are deficient in copper, a bioavailable form of copper that your body can easily assimilate is found in oysters (fresh or canned). If you're lacking zinc, regularly snacking on pumpkin seeds or adding some to your daily smoothie is a great idea. If your body is deficient in iron, zinc, or trace minerals, try eating more red meat (beef, bison, elk, goat, lamb, or venison) since meat is high in the bioavailable heme iron.

In addition to considering bioavailability, you must be aware that some nutrients require the presence of *other* nutrients to be properly absorbed—also known as **nutrient synergy**. This is why it's important that you incorporate fruit into your daily diet since your body requires vitamin C to properly absorb iron from your food.

As an example, I was taking a capsule form of stinging nettle every day to try to increase my iron levels. But because it wasn't giving me enough of the right kind of iron, and I wasn't pairing it with something like rose hips or kiwi for vitamin C, it wasn't doing much to help me. The real problem was that I was deficient in the right *minerals* my body needed to move the iron to the right place.

While vitamin C makes you think of the taste of fresh citrus, vitamin D reminds you of the sun's warmth on your skin. You absorb vitamin D when you are outside in the sun between April and October (in the Northern Hemisphere). Your body needs enough vitamin D in order to absorb vitamin A, vitamin K, and all the B vitamins. Being out in the sunshine is the absolute best method for getting your vitamin D intake (Srivastava, 2021).

If you're Caucasian, you need to spend 5-30 minutes in the sunlight without sunscreen during the brightest part of the day (10 a.m. to 3 p.m.) every day in order to create enough vitamin D inside your body. If you are Hispanic, Black, or have a more melanated complexion, you need to spend even more time in the sun during peak hours for your body to make adequate vitamin D (Dawson-Hughes, 2004). Typically, 30-45 minutes should be enough time for your body to create your needed amount of vitamin D. Any less than the minimum amount of time (for either group), and you will need to consider supplementation.

As a general suggestion, I tell people to be out in the sun for 20 minutes without sunscreen, which has been a good measure for getting enough sun exposure to produce sufficient levels of vitamin D and feel its benefits. It is also the perfect amount of time to get outside and take a walk, improving your vitamin D levels, getting your daily exercise, and supporting your lymphatic system.

If you need to be outdoors for a short period of time for less than an hour on any given day (picking tomatoes in your garden or taking a walk after lunch), it's unnecessary to slather on sunscreen, in my opinion. Normally, I only put sunscreen on my body if I'm going to be out in the garden for several hours or if I'm at the beach.

The problem for me (and millions of other folks who live in the Northern Hemisphere) is that we can only absorb sufficient vitamin D when the sun is at about a 45-50 degree angle to the earth. This means nearly 6 months out of the year, even at high noon, we can't make enough vitamin D in our skin from sun exposure. This is where knowing which foods are naturally high in vitamin D (like liver and oily fish) is very beneficial.

Although you ideally get your vitamin D from sun exposure, it's okay (and sometimes necessary) to supplement with vitamin D in the winter months, especially if you live in the North. Vitamin D can also be found in edible mushrooms, but taking a supplement is likely easier than eating a pound of mushrooms every day. Sufficient vitamin D intake is crucial to bone health, as it allows for calcium absorption and promotes a strong immune system (National Institute of Arthritis and Musculoskeletal and Skin Diseases, 2023). Vitamin D deficiency is linked to anxiety, depression, fibromyalgia, a poorly functioning immune system, and more.

Don't discount the importance of sunlight! You're basically a plant that walks and talks.

Even if you're trying your hardest to eat a high-quality, healthy diet and get outdoors, you may still end up needing a little help. This is why I don't want you to discount the idea of seeing a doctor, as they can provide you with the necessary blood tests to figure out which nutrient (or lack thereof) is causing your current problem. Once you know where the problem lies, you can figure out which foods will help you increase the amount of that nutrient in your body.

Supplementing with a capsule form of synthetic vitamins or minerals should be a last resort, only taken if you realize that your diet or lifestyle is incapable of meeting your body's needs. Again, that's the sort of decision that needs to be informed by having a blood test done to see your nutrient levels.

Don't think you'll find good-quality supplements at Walmart or another big box store because you won't, no matter how fancy the brand's label is. Such supplements are mostly worthless because they are often not in a bioavailable form, not formulated at an effective concentration, or contain filler ingredients that hinder the supplement's effectiveness. Cheap vitamins are expelled almost entirely in your urine (Guo, 2021), meaning your money is quite literally being flushed down the drain.

You can buy specialized "whole food vitamin" supplements online, which are going to be a better choice than store-bought options if you're intent on taking a daily multivitamin. However, since most vitamins remain in your system for around 24-36 hours, you have plenty of time to get most of your nutrition directly from your new, well-balanced diet or the addition of a vitamin-packed daily smoothie.

The human body evolved to extract what it needs from what we eat. There weren't herds of multivitamins roaming the plains for us to hunt 10,000 years ago. Food truly is your best source of nutrition and your most effective medicine when you know what foods to eat.

Chapter 5: Your Food, Your Medicine

Prevention is the best form of treatment you can give to your body. Eating right, getting a balance of food-based vitamins and minerals in your diet, practicing proper sleep hygiene, and exercising at least a little bit each day (especially if it involves being outdoors) can keep you healthier than someone who isn't practicing these simple tips. Taking health-oriented, preventative steps also reduces the amount of inflammation you experience in your body. Yes, there are herbs that can help with inflammation, but wouldn't it be better to not develop it in the first place?

This doesn't mean you can never have a piece of pizza or a root beer float; you just have to accept that eating these sorts of things every day as part of your regular diet is doing your body exponential harm, especially when done over the course of many years.

You're never deficient in herbs, but you CAN be deficient in vitamins and minerals. Your diet, the food you eat every single day, is the most important part of your life to focus on to improve your overall health and well-being. But how?

Eat the rainbow!

Remember ROY G. BIV? Take a moment to be a kid again and go watch the song on YouTube from They Might Be Giants.

Here's a basic breakdown of what the colors of your plant-derived foods indicate in terms of nutrition:

RED: Apples, cranberries, cherries, raspberries, tomatoes, watermelon, peppers, and more—red fruits and vegetables are often high in vitamin A, vitamin C, and potassium.

ORANGE: Apricots, cantaloupe, oranges, carrots, sweet potatoes, winter squash, and more—orange fruits and vegetables are often high in vitamin A, vitamin C, vitamin K, and potassium.

YELLOW: Bananas, lemons, peaches, pineapples, potatoes, squash, and more—yellow fruits and vegetables are often high in vitamin A, vitamin C, vitamin B3, beta carotene, niacin, and potassium.

GREEN: Apples, limes, pears, bok choy, broccoli, collard greens, cucumbers, kale, lettuce, spinach, culinary herbs, and more—green fruits, vegetables, and herbs are often high in vitamin A, vitamin C, vitamin E, vitamin K, calcium, folate, iron, magnesium, and potassium. Green is also the color of most early spring wild plants, such as amaranth, bittercress, dandelion greens, lamb's quarters, stinging nettles, and more. (Sometimes green foods are bitter, and that's a good thing!)

BLUE: Aronia berries, blueberries, grapes, prunes, eggplant, blue potatoes, and more—blue fruits and vegetables are often high in vitamin C, vitamin K, vitamin B6, vitamin B12, and manganese.

Indigo and Violet (a.k.a. Purple): Blackberries, black currants, grapes, serviceberries, black beans, purple cabbage, purple potatoes, and more—purple fruits and vegetables are often high in vitamin A, vitamin C, vitamin K, anthocyanins (Khoo et al., 2017), and antioxidants.

Don't forget that in addition to vitamins and minerals, you get **fiber** from all the fruits and vegetables you eat. Fiber helps your stomach feel full, which helps prevent you from overeating (and thus, helps you lose weight!). Additionally, fiber helps aid digestion, helps prevent constipation (you'll never poop if you don't eat enough fiber), helps prevent heart disease, and helps reduce inflammation.

The part of fruit most people love is the sugar. When you were a kid (or if you have a kid, you may know this), did you want the apple *juice* or the whole apple? The apple juice is sweeter, right? The apple is pulverized and squeezed of all its liquid, which is then boiled and filtered (and sometimes even sweetened) to make the sugary sweet juice that you can drink.

After drinking the juice, your body feels good for a little while, getting a quick hit of sugar and carbohydrates, which fuel energy levels. Your blood sugar rises, and your insulin increases. But shortly after, you feel hungry again, and your energy starts to disappear. So you drink more juice! This does not satiate you for long; you feel hungry again, just like before. Your blood sugar also rises again. If you're diabetic, you know this is something you're supposed to avoid, or at least only have such foods and drinks in moderation.

But when you eat the apple itself, you get to eat the sugary juices surrounded by the pulp (the part of the apple that contains the fiber) and the skin, the way nature intended you to eat it. This way, the fiber slows down the digestion of the sugars in the apple, resulting in a much lower, more manageable blood sugar spike than simply drinking the juice alone. It's almost always preferable that you eat fruits and vegetables in their whole form rather than drinking them as a juice, which robs you of the best part—the fiber.

In short, you're going to get the highest percentage of your required vitamins, minerals, nutrients, and fiber from foods that grow from the ground. While there are some shortcuts, like juices and smoothies, they are not always your best option, since eating the whole fruit or vegetable often extracts more of its benefits. By eating the rainbow, you get the fiber your body needs to function properly—aiding digestion, regulating blood sugar levels, and promoting a feeling of fullness (Brock, 2024).

Chapter 6: Wild Harvesting in Your Own Backyard

Foraging for wild foods is one of my favorite pastimes and my preferred method of feeding myself and my family whenever possible. It's taken me over 18 years of dabbling and learning from the internet, books, and personal experience to become confident in my foraging. Don't be upset if all you are comfortable foraging for right now are some dandelion greens and red clover blossoms. There's a whole world of food out in your backyard; you've got plenty of time to discover one plant at a time.

This isn't a foraging book. I have written books about foraging, and I've filmed hundreds of hours of foraging content that you can watch for free on my social media. But in the interest of offering you a place to start, I'd like to give you a list of my personal favorite foods to forage (SO FAR). I say "so far" because I usually end up tasting a new plant at least twice every year, so my palate is ever-expanding.

Some of my favorite plants have medicinal properties and can be prepared as a medicine (meaning you would prepare them differently to make medicine than you would to cook them). But everything here tastes good either raw or sautéed in a little grass-fed butter.

These are the plants I forage and eat most often:

- Amaranth (*Amaranthus spinosus*)—primarily the leaves before the plant goes to seed
- Black nightshade berries (*Solanum nigrum*)—not to be confused with deadly nightshade**
- Blueberries and huckleberries (*Vaccinium spp.*)
- Burdock root (*Arctium lappa*)—when I can find enough
- Chickweed (*Stellaria media*)
- Dandelion (*Taraxacum officinale*) greens
- Evening primrose (*Oenothera biennis*) roots
- Galinsoga (*Galinsoga parviflora*) leaves
- Greenbriar (*Smilax rotundifolia*) tips—the tip of the vine plus the first few leaves when soft and succulent
- Lamb's quarters (*Chenopodium album*) leaves
- Purslane (*Portulaca oleracea*) leaves
- Queen Anne's lace (*Daucus carota*) roots**
- Red clover (*Trifolium pratense*) flowers
- Stinging nettle (*Urtica dioica*) leaves
- Strawberries (*Fragaria spp.*) fruit and leaves
- Sweet cicely (*Myrrhis odorata*) stems—as a raw snack in spring**
- Violet (*Viola spp.*) leaves and flowers
- Wood sorrel (*Oxalis acetosella*)
- Yellow dock (*Rumex crispus*) leaves

- Various wild mushrooms:
- Black trumpets (*Craterellus cornucopioides*)
- Red chanterelles (*Cantharellus cinnabarinus*)**
- Chicken of the woods (*Laetiporus spp.*)**

****This plant has deadly lookalikes, so you need to study carefully to be certain of identification before consuming!**

As far as mushrooms go, the part of the mushroom you see growing above the ground (or other growing surface) is called the "fruiting body" of the mushroom. This is the part you eat. The mushroom's "roots" are called mycelium and can extend deeper into the earth than what you see growing above the ground. The mycelium of a mushroom can be hundreds of feet wide, but you'll only see a few little mushrooms growing from organic materials or the ground.

If you're harvesting wild mushrooms that you are certain you identified correctly, please use a knife to cut the stem just at the level of the soil (or growing surface) rather than pulling them up or out. Doing so will keep the mycelium intact so the fungus can grow more fruiting bodies again.

I recommend you look up each of the previously listed plants in a book, on Google, or on your plant-identifying app and familiarize yourself with them. My other book, *Forage and Heal: Discovering Plant Identification, Black Walnuts, and Nature's Healing Power*, can be of help to you in learning more about some of the aforementioned plants as well. These plants grow abundantly in North America, particularly in the Northeastern region. They are also a critical source of micronutrients and microdoses of minerals, which are all critical to cellular function inside your body.

While I agree that the majority of our vitamins, minerals, and general nutritive intake should be derived from the whole foods we eat, I am no stranger to taking supplements when necessary.

Although I eat an incredibly nutrient-dense diet over the course of the year, I cook almost exclusively with cast iron, I have meat regularly, and I drink well water that comes out with an orange tint to it because of its iron content, I still wound up with iron-deficiency anemia. I'm currently using supplementation and herbs to bring my levels back into balance. To learn more about treating iron deficiency from an herbalist's perspective, you can watch my short video on just that (linked in the Additional Resources section at the end of the book).

Due to various reasons, mostly having to do with the way agriculture has been practiced over the past 100 years or so, most people are incapable of getting enough magnesium in their diet. Other nutrients that are frequently found to be deficient are calcium, copper, zinc, and sometimes iron (Cazzola et al., 2020). Because of this, supplementation may become necessary to get all the vitamins and minerals our bodies need to function properly and optimally in the event we can't get them through the foods we eat.

Do the best you can with what you have available to you. If you can eat some of the dandelion or wood sorrel growing in your backyard but have to buy all your vegetables from the canned food aisle, that's a perfect start. If you have 50 acres of land to forage and plenty of time to pick and preserve your harvest, do that. Every little thing you can do to supplement or replace the Standard American Diet with whole food sources that will nourish the cells in your body is a win for you, no matter how small!

Chapter 7: What About Meat?

Humans evolved by eating meat, especially cooked meat and the marrow from inside the bones (Pobiner, 2013). Your canine teeth are proof of that. Moreover, our brains developed from eating animal fats. Over time, eating meat (as well as a wide array of plants) led to the evolution of our species as a whole.

In terms of composition, "Meat and marrow are calorie-dense resources with essential amino acids and micronutrients (Milton, 1999, as cited in Pobiner, 2013), and aquatic fauna offer resources rich in nutrients needed for brain growth (e.g., Broadhurst et al., 2002, as cited in Pobiner, 2013)." For the role they play in our development and general health, I suggest everyone eat meat when they can find a high-quality and ethically sourced supply.

You don't have to eat meat every day to reap the nutritional benefits of having it in your diet. Vegans and vegetarians, however, do have a harder time getting enough bioavailable B12, iron, and zinc into their bodies due to their dietary restrictions.

Needless to say, you have the right to choose what foods you do and do not eat. But a well-balanced diet includes meat, and without that source of vitamins and minerals, you're going to have a harder time making sure your body is not deficient in some form of vital nutrition.

Carnitine is a component of red meat (mainly found in beef and lamb). It's also naturally created in the human liver when a person is eating a complete and balanced diet. Getting sufficient carnitine can help reduce the development of Alzheimer's disease, improve heart health, mitigate fatigue, prevent unwanted substances from building up inside your mitochondria (helping your cells get rid of waste), and improve sperm count in men.

I personally dealt with iron-deficiency anemia in late 2024, despite the fact that I had been cooking exclusively in cast iron pans for over ten years and eating many various fruits, vegetables, herbs, and seeds that are high in iron (dandelion greens, dried apricots, spinach, hemp seeds, pumpkin seeds, etc.). During my journey to find a solution, I found a supplement called Hema-Plex that started to help me, but my anemia-related issues persisted.

Eventually, in a last-ditch effort to resolve them, I tried eating liver and onions for the first time. I sautéed a slice of beef liver in my cast iron pan with a big pat of grass-fed butter and half of a sweet white onion. When it was cooked, I picked up a piece of liver and onion in one bite and started chewing.

My mouth exploded with joy! The flavor was not bad at all. Although the texture was a little spongy, it was like my body was screaming MORE, MORE! So I started eating a piece of liver every night as part of my dinner. After about 30 days of doing this, I reduced it to eating liver and onions once a week. I'm feeling SO much better now. To our grandparents who loved this dish, you were right!

As far as sourcing meat, I do have some suggestions:

To preface, I do not support factory farming. I acknowledge you have to buy whatever food your wallet allows you to purchase. But whenever possible, I urge you to support a small local farm. Buying meat that will support your nutritional intake isn't always as simple as driving to the nearest grocery store. If you can afford to buy a higher quality of meat, such as from animals that were raised ethically and sustainably on a local small farm, I highly recommend you do so.

To me, any farm under 200 acres is a small farm; that's still a ton of land. If you cannot buy from a local small farm, I'd be willing to wager there is a farmers market or local CSA you can order meat from. Heck, you may even have a neighbor raising a few head of beef cattle that could sell you half a cow. Do you know how much money you save when you buy half a cow upfront? Yeah, it's probably going to run you around $2,000. But that $2,000 will feed you and your family for almost a *year* on local pasture-raised meat. (Just store it in the freezer until you're ready to cook it.)

I like being able to go to a farm and pet the cow on the head. I want to know that his name is Bart. I want to see that Bart had a really nice life grazing grass, frolicking in the sun, and sleeping under the stars before he was slaughtered carefully and swiftly to be harvested for his meat. Bart was a happy cow, and happy cows are *delicious*.

If you don't know, CSA stands for **Community-Supported Agriculture**. The basic premise is that you pay the farmer around $600 in March or April, and he uses that money to buy seeds, supplies, and whatever else he may need to run his farm. Then, starting in May or June, you get about six solid months of a share of their harvest each week. Many farms (including fruit, vegetable, and meat farms) offer this option. Whichever type you're looking for, just Google "meat CSA," "organic vegetable CSA," etc., and your zip code. Get to know the vendors at your local farmer's market. Once you taste the difference, you'll never go back.

It's worth every penny if you don't have land to farm yourself. It gives you high-quality, farm-fresh food without the middleman (i.e., the grocery store). Not only do you get fresher food, but your money goes straight into the pocket of the farmer rather than some corporate bureaucrat. Even if you can't afford to join a CSA, do your best to find a local small farm near you that you can buy food from. The key is local; the less distance your food has to travel to get to you, the fresher (and usually better) it's going to taste.

Sometimes you can find a small farm that you can volunteer at in exchange for a share of their harvest. Or if you're adventurous, you could even get a job as a farmhand. I went on that adventure for 9 years, and it completely changed my life and my appreciation of food.

There are thousands of resources on how to grow your own vegetables, so I'm not going to talk about that here. What I will say is if you have a space to do so (whether that's a garden in the ground or just a pot on your back steps that you can grow a tomato plant in), DO IT. YouTube is a great free resource that can assist you in starting to grow your own food. Nothing in this world tastes better than food you grew, gathered, hunted, or otherwise made yourself.

Please don't let your inability to grow or raise your own food stop you from eating healthful meals. Simply making the choice to buy fresh (or frozen) produce and the highest quality meats from the best quality sources you can afford is going to help you make the best meals you can. It's more beneficial to opt for whole food options when you can rather than to worry about whether your chicken came from a regenerative farm versus a conventional one.

The important thing is to focus on eating the highest quality foods you can afford to put into your body rather than letting your stomach be filled with nutrient-lacking foods. Think of what your ancestors would have eaten only two hundred years ago and work from there.

Chapter 8: Changing Your Diet, Healing Your Gut

If you deal with a bloated belly, diarrhea, constipation, or any other unpleasant symptom every time you eat a certain food, it may be time for you to re-evaluate its place in your diet. To help you narrow down what foods may be causing you issues, this chapter includes a list of some of the most common allergens of our time. These allergens, when left unchecked, can compromise your gut health and worsen other allergies or chronic conditions you may be experiencing.

Your body is different from my body, and I probably have some allergies or aversions that you don't have. But it is possible you have some of the same allergies as me, since they're fairly common. For instance, I generally stay grain-free because most grains that can be found in the United States are either wheat or a relative of wheat, and my body has difficulty processing gluten.

I also find it important to note that many grain crops are sprayed with pesticides on large-scale "factory farms" where it's unfeasible to use natural methods of pest control. When you grow a hundred acres of the exact same plant all in one space, whatever insect or fungus has evolved to eat that one plant has a smorgasbord to dine on unless you spray the crop with pesticide or fungicides. Hence why large-scale monocropping necessitates the use of pesticides.

While produce covered in pesticide residue doesn't immediately harm humans, over time it can build up in your system (and especially in children). The resulting internal pesticide buildup can cause a higher sensitivity to other foods and pollens, resulting in higher allergic reactions overall (Buralli et al., 2020).

I have a negative reaction to glyphosate and other pesticides, so I avoid them whenever possible. The second farm I ever worked on was purportedly an organic farm. While working, I was given pumpkin seeds to plant, which were coated in some kind of shiny blue stuff. Despite wearing plastic gloves, the blue stuff made contact with my skin, causing me to become dizzy and see spots. Similarly, the last time I used Roundup, spraying weeds in the cracks on my mother's patio, I became dizzy and lightheaded shortly after.

I have enough personal experience with pesticides to never want to touch them again, outside of a few organic ones like BT (Bacillus thuringiensis, a bacteria that kills certain pests) and diatomaceous earth. However, I've recently had surprisingly good results by simply choosing to weed less often. Many of the common garden "weeds" are not only edible but also make excellent trap crops, enticing the local insects to eat them instead of my beloved vegetables.

It is possible to grow without major pesticide use; some farms are beginning to do this on a large scale, which gives me hope for the future. Until there comes a time when this is more widely practiced, I am mindful of the foods I eat, especially the ones that may have been treated with pesticides.

<u>Common food allergens I do not eat and why:</u>

- **Wheat/gluten-containing grains**: I avoid these partly because of farming practices, partly because I bloat up like a balloon when I eat them, and because I feel better when I don't have them. Wheat is one of the most common allergens in the United States today, mainly due to the fact that the Department of Agriculture changed the type of wheat we grow here in the U.S. in the 1950s. They started marketing it before testing what kind of (negative) effects the new strain would have on people who consumed it (Davis, 2011/2019, pp. 23–24). Have you ever noticed that the number of people who are allergic to wheat has increased since the 60s? This is why. Since it's difficult to find unadulterated wheat, I prefer to avoid it completely. You can dive deeper into the more nuanced reasons not to eat gluten by reading Dr. William Davis' book, *Wheat Belly*.

- **Cow dairy products** (aside from butter): As a substitute, I eat goat and sheep cheese and milk. The only cow dairy I can safely have is a little bit of hard Parmesan cheese or a small amount of mozzarella. Dairy is one of the most common allergens in the United States (Warren et al., 2022). Lactose intolerance is incredibly prevalent across the globe because children in most cultures stop drinking milk by the age of 5. Europeans developed the ability to digest lactose as a survival mechanism during times of death and famine, such as during the Black Plague (Thompson, 2012). If you could digest milk, it served as an additional food source for you during times when food was scarce. However, people who share DNA with other genetic regions generally lack the digestive enzymes necessary for processing cow milk beyond their 20s. As a result, much of the population is unable to properly digest cow dairy, leading to varying degrees of milk intolerance and allergy.

- **Peanut butter**: This makes me cry and shake my fist at the world. I LOVE peanut butter. But even the healthy stuff that's only made with peanuts and salt is subject to mold toxicity. This is because it's impossible for companies to check every single peanut for signs of mold before they are ground up (by the millions) into butter. The chances that these peanuts have traces of mold on them are actually significantly higher than you may think. Then, the butter is put into containers and left to sit in the cupboard for ages. Even if you are not deathly allergic to peanuts, as some people are, lesser peanut allergies are something to be aware of. For me, it causes the same rash as cane sugar does. Occasionally, I'll deal with the rash just to get a taste of the sweet peanut ambrosia I love so much. If you do want to keep peanut butter in your diet, it's a good idea to either grow and make your own or avoid it whenever possible. Unfortunately, the risk of mold is pretty high in all store-bought nut butters.

- **Soy products**: I occasionally make an exception when I have small amounts of properly fermented soy sauce. Here, I'm referring to the kind you can find only in an authentic Asian food store. Other than that, soy generally makes me bloated and gassy. Soy is one of the most pesticide-laden crops in America, according to the USDA's National Agricultural Statistics Service (2024). Additionally, unfermented soy contains isoflavones, which are phytoestrogens that can potentially cause hormone imbalances in estrogen-sensitive individuals (The Nutrition Source, 2018).

When originally writing this book, there was one more common culprit present in the above list, which I have recently found a solution to. **Cane sugar** used to be a food allergy for me, which sucked! Any time I ate anything made with cane sugar, white sugar, or molasses, I would get a wildly itchy rash on my inner elbow. No sugar, no rash. For a long time, I stuck with honey and maple syrup as my go-to sweeteners to avoid said rash.

I also experimented with beet sugar, coconut sugar, date sugar, monk fruit extract, allulose, and stevia. Beet sugar was a win; it didn't cause any reaction and is a decent substitute for sugar in recipes. Coconut sugar was hit or miss (sometimes still causing the rash), so I got cautious with using it. Date sugar is delicious and contains fiber. Monk fruit extract is extremely sweet, so it should be used sparingly. Allulose is a blood sugar-friendly option but not quite as sweet, so recipes required tweaking. And stevia? It's SUPER sweet, so be careful.

Here's the exciting part: I very recently healed my cane sugar allergy. I am stoked that I no longer have to stress about consuming tiny amounts of sugar when I'm out and want to treat myself. Best of all, I know what I did to fix it. If you're dealing with some weird allergy that won't budge, the solution I found may be worth trying. I've taken this supplement every afternoon for the past 3 months, taking it for about 12 weeks before it began to fully work its magic: Silver Fern™ Postbiotic+ (Link in Resources). It smells bad and does not taste much better, but I DO NOT CARE. I pour a packet into a small glass of water (half-full is plenty) and chug it after lunch. It's worth every penny.

Although I've found a solution to my sugar allergy, I still only indulge in it sparingly. Just because I am not having a physical reaction I can observe doesn't mean it's not having a negative impact on my gut, skin, and general health. Dietary sugars (especially refined sugars) remain a major contributor to insulin resistance and low-grade chronic inflammation (Ma et al., 2022), both of which I want to avoid. As the famous saying goes, "Moderation in all things."

The Complications from a Poor/Pro-Inflammatory Diet

Did you know that food allergies and nutritional deficiencies can greatly exacerbate conditions such as attention deficit/hyperactivity disorder and autism spectrum disorder? Although more research is needed to fully understand the correlation between the two, recent studies have "found a significant and positive association between common allergic conditions, including food allergy, respiratory allergy, and skin allergy, and ADHD in children" (Xu et al., 2022). Similar conclusions were reached when researching the association between food allergies and other allergic conditions with ASD in children (Xu et al., 2018).

Incidentally, a whole foods diet (and the other recommendations in this book, such as supplementation and exercise) is the best option you will find for managing symptoms caused by these conditions. If you or your child are dealing with ADHD, I suggest you get the book *Finally Focused* by Bill Gottlieb and James Greenblatt. It goes over diet changes and supplementation specific to treating ADHD in much greater detail than you will find in this book.

There is now scientific evidence that suggests Alzheimer's disease is a form of type 3 diabetes (Douda, 2017). The prevalence of type 2 diabetes and insulin resistance in a population that grows more obese with each generation has encouraged scientists to look into the connection between Alzheimer's and diabetes. I do know that those who suffer from Alzheimer's or dementia-related symptoms are typically dealing with chronic problems that developed from as early a time as their 30s.

My grandmother developed dementia late in her life. The last time I saw her was when she and my grandfather visited me after the birth of my first child. I was devastated to see how little she was able to do on her own, the woman who had helped raise me. In one breath she offered to watch the baby while I did some grocery shopping and simultaneously asked where the kitchen was for the third time when she was standing right beside it.

My great-grandfather, her father, had dementia as well. Knowing that dementia runs in my family, I am taking preventative measures *now* to avoid that fate for myself. If you have a family history of dementia or Alzheimer's, I suggest you seriously consider following the dietary advice in this book. I would rather never eat pizza or cake again than succumb to dementia, unable to remember my loved ones or take care of myself when I am older.

If all this sounds overwhelming right now, let me simplify it for you: if it grows in the ground and isn't toxic, it's probably good to eat. If it eats the things that grow in the ground, it's probably good to eat. Michael Pollan said it best: "Eat food, not too much, mostly plants" (2008, p. 1). To learn more about nutrition, I highly recommend Paul Bergner's book, *The Healing Power of Minerals, Special Nutrients, and Trace Elements.* Although it was published in the 90s, it remains relevant, and I reference it regularly.

Know that your diet affects EVERY part of your body, whether you like it or not. This is not limited to your physical body but includes your mental and emotional health as well (as discussed in Chapters Thirty-Seven and Thirty-Eight). If you know or suspect that you're allergic or intolerant to a certain food, try eliminating it to see if you feel better when not eating it. If your body, mind, and emotional state feel better by eating nutrient-rich foods and avoiding common allergens, even for just one week, think of how amazing you're going to feel when you eat this way ALL THE TIME!

Chapter 9: The *Easiest* Whole Meal

Now that you know what sort of foods you should be eating, how do you put them all together? There are thousands of health coaches out there, and even ChatGPT can write an entire meal plan for you. But let's keep it simple! I've been cooking daily for the last 25 years; I can promise you that making quick, easy meals that taste great just takes a little bit of practice.

I always suggest you grow herbs whenever possible, whether they're in a pot on your porch or in garden beds. Snip off a few pieces of ANY cooking herb (oregano, parsley, sage, thyme, etc.) and add to any meal that you think it complements well. The extra flavor and vitamins will be much appreciated by your body as well as your taste buds.

What follows are a couple bare-bones recipes that you can rinse and repeat as often as you like. You can use the first one to cook a variety of different vegetables and experiment with different meats too. Instead of ground beef one night, you could chop up some leftover roast chicken or thin round steak. Any pound of any meat will do for this. The same goes for vegetables (except things you only want to eat fresh, like lettuce or radishes).

The second recipe is great when the weather's cold outside. Most farmers have more butternut squash than they know what to do with come October, so you should be able to get quite a few inexpensively. They usually store well for at least a few months, giving you plenty of time to work this recipe into your rotation.

To walk through it with me step-by-step, you can follow along with my video tutorial for this recipe (linked in the Additional Resources section at the end of the book).

Note: The best possible ingredients you can buy are preferred. If you can afford to buy organic or pasture-raised items at the store, do so. If you can only afford conventional foods, make sure you stick to whole foods like fruits, vegetables, meats, nuts, and seeds.

Rainbow Stir-Fry Recipe

1 lb meat (ground or chopped)

Either 2 potatoes, washed and chopped (not peeled), OR 1 cup of cooked wild rice

Whatever vegetables (fresh or frozen) you have on hand, chopped into bite-sized chunks (beets, broccoli, cabbage, garlic, kale, mushrooms, onions, peppers, squash, tomatoes, etc.)

2 Tbsp. butter or bacon fat

Salt, pepper, and any herbs or spices you enjoy

Instructions:

Heat a cast iron skillet on medium heat. Add the butter (or bacon fat) to your skillet. Once the butter is melted, add the onions (and potatoes if you are adding them) and sauté for five to ten minutes. Then, add the remaining vegetables and cook for another five minutes. Once the veggies have begun to soften, add the meat and use a wooden spatula to break it up and move it around the pan. Sprinkle your herbs and spices over everything and continue to cook until all the meat is browned and the vegetables have softened.

If you chose rice instead of potatoes, add it to the pan and stir. Salt as desired and serve in bowls to eat. Any foraged foods or wild-infused vinegar may be a nice addition to this. Get creative!

Harvest Soup Recipe

2 Tbsp butter or bacon fat

1 onion, chopped

1 apple, chopped

2 celery sticks, chopped

2-3 cups of peeled and cubed winter squash (butternut, pumpkin, etc.)

3 cloves garlic, chopped

1 1/2 cups chicken or vegetable bone broth

Parsley, thyme, sage, or any other herbs you have on hand (fresh or dried)

1 tsp paprika powder

½ tsp black pepper

1 Tbsp sea salt

Optional: ¼ tsp cayenne pepper

1 cup of sour cream (I use Lactaid brand)

Instructions:

In a Dutch oven or other large pot, sauté your onions in butter for 3-4 minutes until they begin to turn clear. Then, add the broth and all other ingredients—except the herbs, seasoning, and sour cream—and bring to a boil.

Turn down to low heat and simmer for 30 minutes. Turn the heat off or to very low. After the vegetables have cooked through, add your seasoning.

Use an immersion blender to blend the soup into a smooth consistency, then add the sour cream and stir it in until well incorporated.

Turn the heat back on low and allow to cook for 5 more minutes, stirring occasionally. Taste the soup and adjust the seasoning to your liking.

Being able to cook for yourself is an essential life skill that many people have either forgotten or never learned thanks to the modern industrial food complex and the advent of ready-made frozen dinners. However, with a little practice (and probably an unhealthy addiction to the recipe side of Pinterest), you can learn to satisfy your cravings with foods that aren't pumped full of preservatives and ingredients you can't pronounce.

If you're looking for more recipes, I have many more available on my social media, in my Forage and Heal book, and in my Wildcrafted Eats course (all linked at the end of the book in the Additional Resources section). It's taken me years to become a fantastic cook with much time, practice, and experimentation. If you can follow a good recipe and use herbs to enhance your dish, you'll have mastered the skill in no time!

Chapter 10: Hydration

I cannot stress this enough: DRINK WATER. Drink enough water every day! By the time your body signals that it's thirsty, you may already be up to 2% dehydrated (The Health Sciences Academy, 2021). It's important to drink enough water throughout the day. I mean actual water (or plain seltzer is okay, since it's just water with bubbles added to it). Not soda, not Gatorade, not Pedialyte, not Red Bull, and not Brawndo—these are not what your body needs. Brawndo is *not* what plants crave. Remember, you're basically a plant that can walk and talk. You need sunlight, food, and WATER.

You can find a good guide on recommended daily water intake on Harvard's website, The Nutrition Source. Each person's daily water needs will be slightly different, based on their weight, metabolism, and level of activity (Oliveira, 2025). Your big bear of a 6'4" uncle Bob is going to need a few gallons of water (and a little salt) to stay hydrated during your family soccer game, while your brother, who is only 5'7" with a physique like Spider-Man, will do well on considerably less.

How do you know you're properly hydrated? Your pee will be light yellow.

Dark yellow pee means you're dehydrated. Orange pee means you're dangerously dehydrated (unless it's caused by a supplement or medication you're taking). Your pee may also be darker after you take a vitamin capsule.

With vitamin capsules, you typically pee out most of the vitamins before they can be properly absorbed, so they're not doing you much good. The majority of B vitamins, including B1, B2, B3, B5, B6, B7, and B12, are among the water-soluble vitamins you are likely to lose in your urine, partly because you're getting them from food sources and partly because the multivitamin is giving your body more than it needs.

If your pee is clear, you're probably drinking *too much* water. If your pee is tinged with red or pink, either you ate beets recently or you could have blood in your urine. If it's not from eating beets, call your doctor to get that checked out.

If you find yourself peeing a lot, more frequently than what you're used to (and it's not because you're drinking nettle tea), talk with your doctor and get your kidney function checked. Abnormally frequent urination and urgency can be a sign of a problem.

I always start my morning by drinking a glass of water with a slice of lemon squeezed into it. I used to drink cold water upon waking, but I recently read that drinking warm or hot water can wake up your gut and encourage your body to relax. I began drinking warm water (not boiling, just warm from the tap) in the mornings, and it is more relaxing. It also promotes relaxation of the bowels, encouraging a healthy bowel movement in the morning following breakfast (Çalişkan et al., 2016).

I have heard it suggested that you should abstain from drinking water (or any other drink) while eating a meal, as it can dilute your body's naturally produced digestive enzymes. It's up to you; do what's comfortable. I do my best to follow this rule, but I naturally feel like I need to drink more water when I eat, so I take a digestive enzyme capsule to compensate.

I accidentally discovered my favorite beverage about two years ago when I bought a seltzer-making machine (the thing that squirts CO2 into your water to make it bubbly). I bought the "flavor syrup" to make my own flavored seltzer. I realized, however, that I could not find any flavoring options that had naturally occurring sweeteners or flavorings in them. One night, I began to experiment by simply cutting a lime into quarters and squeezing one of them into a glass. I filled the glass with plain seltzer, and HOLY CRAP, it's the best, most refreshing drink I've ever had! My son and I have a glass every night with dinner.

It's exponentially healthier than drinking soda or a bottled seltzer with mystery flavoring, and it fulfills my desire to drink something other than plain water or tea all the time. I wouldn't suggest you drink this all day because too much citrus on your teeth can degrade the enamel over time, but a glass at night should not do any harm. As they say, "All good things in moderation."

Finally, always be sure to take water with you when you leave the house—when you go hiking, to the beach, or anywhere else you go, especially when you go outdoors. Keep water in your vehicle. Have your kids take water to school with them. There's nothing shameful about being hydrated.

Chapter 11: Movement

Moving your body is critical to your health, and it's more than just reaching into the refrigerator for a snack! It's best to acclimate to exercising in some way daily while you're young. If you did not do that when you were a kid, you can at least have your friends or kids go on a walk or easy hike with you once in a while. They may say they don't like it (and you may not like it to start), but once you make it onto a nature trail, feeling the sun and breeze on your skin, I suspect you'll want to get outdoors more and more. Even if you live in an urban area, I encourage you to spend some time every week in your local park.

Personally, I am guilty of not moving my body enough, just as many people are guilty of. I spend far too much time either seated at my computer desk or standing in the kitchen. One key to living a pain-free life is to prioritize moving your body in a myriad of ways on a daily basis. If you want to pretend you're going to the Ministry of Silly Walks on your way from the car into work, that's great! You're moving your body in weird and unusual ways and giving yourself a good laugh at the same time.

We each have to adhere to our own time schedule, managing responsibilities that demand our time and attention. The excuse we all give is "I don't have enough time." In reality, it is more often possible than not to carve out ten minutes of our day to devote to getting up and moving around. And doing so, on a daily basis, helps mitigate the body pain we experience the older we get.

Whether you join a yoga class, follow a few workout videos online, or just go for a 30-minute walk every afternoon, make sure you move your body and get your heart rate up. Regular daily movement can improve digestion, help prevent diverticulitis, reduce bloating after meals, and move lymph through your body (Mayo Clinic Staff, 2023). You don't have to go to the gym and lift weights for an hour to change the way your body feels and looks.

I will mention, however, that lifting weights, even if it's only your own body weight, is necessary for women over 45 to maintain their muscle tone and reduce the prevalence of meno-belly (Chesak, 2024). I encourage you to take a few minutes and look up bodyweight exercises you can do at home on YouTube and try one that looks interesting to you.

Whether you're walking on a walking pad while you watch TV after dinner or lifting weights to train for the Olympics, as long as you're moving your body (in a way that raises your heart rate) for at least 30 minutes a day, you're on your way to maintaining your metabolic health. Ultimately, you want to find an activity that keeps you young and that you enjoy doing.

Chapter 12: Supplementation

If you're over 40, my guess is you're already familiar with, and likely taking, supplements. Are you seeing ads for supplements online? Are you googling your symptoms and trying whatever supplements come up in the search results to see if they'll help you?

I met a woman recently who was taking no fewer than 30 supplements (herbs, vitamins, etc.) as well as a few medications every morning, all at once. When I asked her which ones were helping her symptoms, she honestly didn't know. She was basically throwing "the kitchen sink" at the problem, as many people do in her situation.

Supplementation can certainly help with various issues and deficiencies, but it should be used strategically as part of an overall health plan specific to your body's needs. What I've written in this book is general advice that applies to a majority of people, based on the most common deficiencies I've observed in the people I've worked with. If you want guidance and suggestions that are specific to you, a consultation with an herbalist or naturopath is in order.

Two supplements I want you to consider taking (because getting enough from food-based sources alone is nearly impossible these days) are magnesium and DHA (omega-3s). *[Links in back of book]*

It's exceedingly difficult to get enough magnesium from fruits and vegetables, mainly because the soil in this country has been depleted by over 100 years of unsustainable agricultural practices. Look up how much magnesium you should be getting daily and compare it to how much you are actually getting from the foods you are eating on a regular basis. If you are not getting the specified amount from your diet, this would be an instance to supplement.

I would suggest around 300 mg a day for women and 500 mg a day for men. Be aware that magnesium supplements are harder to absorb than food-based magnesium, so you want to stagger your supplements throughout the day. Take one at noon, another a few hours later, another a few hours after that, etc., until you reach your desired amount. Again, this is a general recommendation for a person who is not on any medications and is not currently taking any kind of magnesium supplement already.

In general, magnesium should be partnered with calcium because you need enough calcium in your body to absorb magnesium and enough magnesium to absorb calcium. However, they need to be taken separately and a few hours apart in order to be properly absorbed. Magnesium is at least partially responsible for a whole host of bodily functions, such as regulating your blood pressure, supporting bone density (reducing the chance of osteoporosis), and helping regulate and balance hormone production (National Institutes of Health, 2022).

Magnesium deficiency can present itself in your body as muscle twitches, poor tolerance of stress, anxiety, depression, insulin resistance, high levels of inflammation, and estrogen dominance or abnormal levels of progesterone. Taking magnesium glycinate, or the even more absorbable magnesium bisglycinate, can result in you getting more consistent and better-quality sleep. It can also help minimize or resolve twitching and restless legs syndrome in many cases (Jadidi et al., 2022).

DHA, or omega-3 fatty acids, is perfectly bioavailable from good-quality fish. However, not only do most of us not include enough fish in our diet, but we now also have to contend with the *quality* of the fish we are able to procure (Horrocks & Yeo, 1999). Unless you are a fisherman or know a good fisherman who will share some of their catch, you'll have to buy your fish from the store like the rest of us.

The grocery store rarely openly discloses whether the fish they're selling you was caught via traditional methods (excellent), nets (okay depending on their practices of throwing back what they don't want), or fishing trawler (the worst, most environmentally destructive method of catching seafood known to man). I try to either eat a can of wild-caught sardines every week or take an algae-based DHA supplement (because where do you think the fish get it from?).

DHA (docosahexaenoic acid) and fish oil can help balance the oils in your body. Did you know that when your skin is dehydrated, sometimes it's not just water you're deficient in? Your body needs oils in your diet to lubricate your skin cells, and incorporating high-quality oils in your diet helps do this. DHA also plays an essential role in our brain development and our nervous system (Swanson et al., 2012). It reduces overall inflammation as well, which can help ease general pain inside your body and specifically endometriosis-related pain.

There is so much more to choosing the right supplements for your personal needs than I can address in a book that's meant to apply to everyone. If the supplements you're currently taking don't seem to be having an effect on your body, I suggest you get some bloodwork or consult with a functional medicine practitioner who can help you figure out exactly which supplements *your* body needs.

It's smarter to seek help from someone knowledgeable about these things than to continue guessing and experimenting on your own body for years with mixed results. Trust me, I know that from experience!

Chapter 13: Sleep

Getting sufficient sleep is critical to your health. Whether you can get to sleep or not is a matter of hormone balance. Since the liver and thyroid significantly affect your hormones, supporting them with the right balance of nutrition will help your sleep A LOT. Your melatonin levels must also be high enough and kick in at the right time of evening for your body to have restful sleep. Not being able to get adequate sleep at night can seriously interfere with all of your bodily systems and make your hormone imbalances worse, causing a vicious cycle of insomnia and fatigue (Kim et al., 2015).

Melatonin is the hormone that your body produces that causes you to fall asleep. You start feeling tired as the daylight fades because your melatonin levels increase as it becomes darker. If you are having difficulty sleeping at night, I do not recommend you take melatonin supplements, at least not until you have tried everything else. (Note: Do not give melatonin to young children! Doing so can interfere with their body's ability to manufacture the hormone on its own over time.)

Instead, try resetting your **circadian rhythm**, the function of your body that causes you to be awake or asleep. If you can manage to, take a 4-5 day period off work and either camp outside or set an alarm so you wake up with the sun in the morning. Then, go to bed shortly after dark. During this time, concentrate on eating natural whole foods and getting the nutrition your body needs. After a week or so of this, your body's circadian rhythm should be reset to its optimal state.

If you do want to try herbs to aid your sleep, you will want to look for **nervine herbs**, which help calm your nervous system. Here, I'm going to give you a few nervine herbs that are commonly used to help aid sleep. Please look more deeply into each of these herbs, as they all have different affinities—treating different types of nervous disorders or reasons for sleeplessness. The below herbs grow readily in most portions of North America, so they should not be difficult to find for sale or grow in your own backyard. There are many more herbs than what I list here; this is just a place for you to get started.

My go-to herbs for sleep, stress, and nerves:

Chamomile (*Matricaria recutita*): This is the general go-to herb for aiding sleep for most Western herbalists. Just know that a single bag of Celestial Seasonings chamomile tea steeped for 5 minutes, while nice, is no substitute for a tablespoon of homegrown chamomile steeped for 30 minutes or more. The stronger infusion will always win! To be taken as a tea or tincture.

Passionflower (*Passiflora incarnata*): This one specifically helps quiet mental chatter. When you can't get your brain to shut the hell up, passionflower may help. To be taken as a tea or tincture.

Wild lettuce (*Lactuca spp.*): Wild lettuce is a hypnotic nervine that specifically helps you fall asleep if the thing that is keeping you awake is physical pain. To be taken as a tincture or boiled down into tar.

Catnip (*Nepeta cataria*): While catnip may make your cat go wild, for a human it serves two amazing purposes: helping you feel sleepy and helping you stop farting. A win for both you and your bedmate! To be taken as a tea.

Milky oats (*Avena sativa*): The sap from this nervine helps people who suffer from mental or physical exhaustion and lack of focus. It is a great daily tonic for those dealing with high stress levels. This is a tincture made from fresh oats (yes, the kind you eat!) with their milky white sap. When oats first form, they are green and soft. If you cut one open, they contain a sap, similar to the white stuff that leaks out of a dandelion stem when you cut it open. Simply harvest the whole oats when they're still in their green stage and make your tincture with the broken pods to capture the sap's stress-relieving properties.

Other herbs you may want to try: California poppy, lavender, skullcap, and Tulsi

The general advice for anyone who has trouble sleeping is to stop eating two hours before you go to bed and stop screen time at least an hour before you go to bed. To end screen time, turn off your TV, stop scrolling your phone, and sit in bed with a book or the person you love and just cuddle up.

You can meditate or listen to binaural beats or sound therapy. Yes, I will use my phone to bring up a sound bath video, but 20 seconds of searching on YouTube isn't the same as mindlessly scrolling through short videos until you pass out. Whatever you can do to lower your cortisol and relax your nervous system in the evening is going to be very beneficial for helping you get a full 7-8 hours of rest. If you have racing thoughts or are worrying about what may happen tomorrow, concentrate on RIGHT NOW. Focus on what you have and where you are. Are you in a bed? Do you have blankets or pillows? Are you warm or cool enough? Is your belly full? Do you have enough fresh air to breathe? You are safe. It's safe to sleep tonight. You are okay for now; tomorrow isn't here yet. You're allowed to rest and recharge. Now, get to sleep!

Chapter 14: What You Wear Matters

Whenever possible, it's best to wear natural fabrics. There was a simple study done in 2020 in which a man buried two pairs of underpants in the ground: one 100% cotton, the other polyester (CottonAustralia, 2020). After 6 months, he dug the area up. Only about half the fabric was present on the cotton underpants, as the rest had composted into the soil. The polyester underwear, on the other hand, looked dirty but was otherwise almost like new.

The cotton decomposed because natural fibers break down over time. As the fabric deteriorated from the changes in soil temperature and moisture, it was also eaten by the various insects, worms, and fungi in the soil. This doesn't happen with polyester, rayon, and other man-made synthetic fabrics.

Did you know that modern humans have the equivalent of a plastic spoon's worth of microplastics inside our bodies (specifically in our brains)? While further research is needed to truly understand this fact's health consequences, it is alarming to see that nanoplastics are invading individual cells and tissues in major organs (LaMotte, 2025). We certainly don't need to add any more microplastics to our bodies by wearing clothes derived from plastics.

Natural fabrics tend to be more expensive, for sure. But they're also better constructed than synthetic fabrics. Yes, they will deteriorate completely if you bury them, but that's because natural fabrics are edible to microorganisms and insects that live in soil. When they're on your body, they're more comfortable and stronger against wear and tear.

Personally, I don't mind spending good money on a piece of clothing that is going to last a long time when properly cared for. I've worn a rayon shirt that I paid a little less for but that tore open after two wears, rendering it useless. Alternatively, it takes months to wear a hole in my wool leggings, which I paid a little more for but have gotten better use out of.

Don't let the price scare you! Think of it this way: Would you rather spend $100 on a shirt that you can wear for 10 years or $10 on a shirt that you can wear for 10 months? If you cannot buy firsthand, natural fabrics, you can check thrift shops or even learn to sew to upcycle old clothing into something new. If you can find (or create) a handmade piece you love, all the better. Then you're paying someone a living wage for an artistic piece you can show off every day to anyone who sees you.

Natural fabrics also allow your skin to BREATHE, and as we know, keeping your skin dry whenever possible is very important. **Breathability**, in reference to clothing, means that the weave is loose enough for air to pass through it to reach your skin. Without breathability, moisture can get trapped in certain areas of your body and encourage bacterial overgrowth, which you want to do everything you can to avoid. My top choices of natural, breathable fabrics are cotton, hemp, linen, and wool.

I love wearing merino wool because while many wool sweaters and socks are itchy or scratchy on my sensitive skin, merino is quite soft and pleasant. It doesn't shed as much as alpaca or angora wool and keeps me warm while letting my skin breathe.

So far, Woolx is my favorite clothing company to buy wool clothing from. I also like Pact for sustainable cotton clothing.

If you've never worn or slept on real linen, you are missing out! Unfortunately, it's a bit difficult to find linen clothing here in the U.S., but I have found quite a few stunning pieces on Etsy. Buying natural fabrics from stores based overseas can also be a viable option to consider, as it's been easier for me to find European-made linen and wool garments than ones made in the U.S.

It has taken me a few years, but I'm now close to having replaced my entire wardrobe with natural fabric clothing. In my experience, natural fabrics are far superior for their composition, quality, lifespan, and breathability. I encourage you to compare the wear (and tear) of natural clothing versus synthetic clothing to see the difference for yourself.

Chapter 15: Hygiene

I don't care how good your hygiene is; there's always something new you can learn. I don't write this chapter to shame anyone. If there are things you read in this chapter that you simply did not know, that's okay! It took me more than half my life to learn all these things. Sometimes your parents aren't capable of teaching you or are too embarrassed to do so.

Many people feel ashamed of their intimate body parts and are afraid to touch them due to some misplaced sense of body negativity. A lot of people feel ashamed of the way their teeth and gums look and refuse to see a dentist because they know that they're supposed to be brushing and flossing, and they simply aren't doing so.

I am writing this section with no shame, no flowery language, and with brutal honesty. What follows are hygiene practices that I learned firsthand, that I wish I had known sooner, and that I am now passing on to you.

Wash Your Hands

I cannot stress this enough; it's so simple. Soap is one of the greatest inventions of man. Use it!

When you go to the store and touch all the things a thousand other people's hands have touched that day (including the virus-laden shopping cart handle), you're exposing yourself to billions of germs. Every time you get home, wash your hands.

I've drilled this into my kids' heads since the day they could walk. When we go into the house from being out ANYWHERE, we wash our hands. If you're out at a library, museum, or shopping all day, wash your hands any time you go to the bathroom.

When you've been out anywhere touching things, wash your hands. I keep unscented hypoallergenic Wet Ones in my vehicle at all times in case I'm out and about and can't get to a sink and soap. Washing your hands is better than using hand sanitizer. Sanitizer is to be used as a last resort when you have no other option, like if you're at a festival and you use the porta-potty and the only way to get your hands clean after you go is to use a pump of sanitizer.

WASH. YOUR. DAMNED. HANDS.

This kills germs and viruses and helps prevent you from putting those germs into your body when you inevitably touch your eye, mouth, nose, or any other part of your body that should not be exposed to germs.

Clean Your Body

Every time you shower, whether that's daily or every few days (ideally at least once a week), wash your body parts with an unscented soap. If you read the ingredients label on your soap and the ingredient "fragrance" is listed, that is not something you want to be putting on your body. Companies hide a LOT of ingredients by using that word—mostly toxic substances that can negatively affect your hormones, make ADHD worse in children, and cause various allergic reactions (Rádis-Baptista, 2023). Please either use unscented soap or soap that's scented with only essential oils.

I've taken a steaming hot shower nearly every day of my adult life. It took my well going dry and having to go nearly four weeks without running water in my home to realize that the reason my back was always itchy was because I was burning off the layer of oil my skin had naturally built up over the day. When I switched to taking a full shower once every *other* day, my skin was fine (or at least a heck of a lot less itchy!). On non-shower days, I do my best to wash up my lady bits before bed. Once the weather warms up, I shower daily because my skin excretes sweat and sebum aplenty, necessitating more frequent washing.

What about deodorant and antiperspirant? I may be in the minority, but I don't like antiperspirant at all. It clogs the pores in your armpits and often contains ingredients that sensitize people's skin, causing allergic reactions and contact dermatitis. After trying out several different natural and homemade deodorant recipes, I have settled on Crystal mineral deodorant. It comes in unscented or sometimes lightly scented liquid forms. It does need to be reapplied a couple times throughout the day, but that's a small price to pay for reducing my exposure to chemicals that could do my body more harm than good.

After you shower and dry off—I don't care what gender you are—go sit somewhere for a few minutes and air yourself out before you get dressed. This is especially important for women because they need to sit spread-eagle (legs spread open) to get airflow in their crotch region. Airflow is ESSENTIAL. Getting proper airflow and airing out "down there" daily plays a big part in helping prevent bacterial vaginosis. If you repeatedly suffer from this condition, you need to pay attention to your diet, make sure you're consuming good probiotics daily (more than just acidophilus), and get good airflow down there.

Also, be aware that if you are sexually active and your partner does not have good genital hygiene, they may be passing bacteria to you during sex, which can cause the infection to keep recurring. My honest recommendation in that case is to have a serious conversation about hygiene with your partner, and if they refuse to change their habits and keep their intimate area clean simply because the bacteria isn't bothering THEM, remove yourself from that relationship.

I can't tell you how many people have asked me how to reduce a boil, pimple, rash, or other blemish "down there." Yeah, you can apply witch hazel to the area to help, but do you know why it helps? Because the astringent nature of witch hazel dries out the skin tissue! Keeping your skin DRY as often as possible is your best defense against overly moist skin problems, as well as helping you avoid yeast infections and bacterial vaginosis.

Change your sheets weekly and your clothing, especially your underwear, daily. Dead skin cells and hair fall off your body every second of every day, not to mention whatever bits of fluid are left behind in your underwear after a trip to the bathroom, no matter how well you wipe. Instead of stewing in your body's own refuse, change into something fresh. Wash your laundry weekly. Make it happen. You'll feel better for it, I promise.

Your Hair—Hygiene and Growth

As far as hair goes, I'll admit that I'm no expert, and I'm still figuring it out. The common consensus is that you're only supposed to wash your hair once a week. If you're like me, only washing once a week will make you look like a greaseball. I wash my hair every three days, and on the days in between, I use The Earthling Co. Dry Shampoo.

Increasing hair growth can be a struggle depending on your hair type. I found success after I started eating beef liver once or twice a week because it increased my copper and iron intake—two minerals that are essential for healthy hair growth (Kil et al., 2013). Silica supplements didn't help me until I started getting enough copper and iron because, without them, my body wasn't able to move the silica to my hair the way it needed to. In terms of hair growth, biotin supplements did not work for me.

If you choose to try eating beef liver to see if it helps your hair grow, which I recommend you do, make sure you give it a few months to see if you notice more growth than you would usually see over a certain amount of time. It's likely that your hair struggles are a bit different than mine in one way or another, but I think almost everyone would benefit from having liver and onions regularly.

Oral Health

Oral health is the health of your mouth: your teeth, gums, lips, etc. I'm not a dentist, but I've had my fair share of dental work. We all know we're supposed to brush our teeth at least twice a day and floss between them at least once a day (Kaloti, 2021). But how many people actually do?

I personally LOVE going to the dentist. I love the feeling of getting my teeth nice and clean and knowing when something is not quite right so I can work on repairing it. I actually *like* the feeling of my gums being massaged and a toothpick getting into the deep crevices that my toothbrush can't reach. But I know not everyone else feels that way.

Many people fear going to the dentist, either due to a past traumatic experience or the fear of being judged for their poor oral health. I'm not here to judge you. I can't even see you. But I will tell you why you should reconsider taking care of your oral health, because it's about SO much more than just having white teeth.

Periodontal (gum) disease and tooth decay have been linked to conditions like diabetes, dementia, heart disease, kidney disease, preterm birth, and cancer (McMains, 2024). Those with poor oral health or gum disease have weaker immune systems than people with good oral health, and as a result, gum disease is also linked to autoimmune disorders like rheumatoid arthritis (Mayo Clinic Staff, 2024). What I'm telling you is that if you don't take care of the inside of your mouth, you risk developing or worsening a whole host of other health problems.

I'm not a fan of fluoride. Fluoride use and ingestion have been linked to lowered IQ, confusion, and Alzheimer's disease. The EPA has even come under serious fire for their part in recommending fluoridated drinking water (Tin, 2024).

In place of fluoride, I much prefer to use and recommend remineralizing powder. So, what's remineralizing powder? It's powdered minerals mixed with a few other ingredients that you brush your teeth with, which helps rebuild the material your teeth are made of. It's made from natural ingredients like bentonite clay, and it doesn't contain all the toxins and soaps that Crest or other commercial toothpastes have. (That's right! Regular toothpaste contains literal SOAP. That's why it gets all foamy inside your mouth.) I've been brushing with remineralizing powder for over two years now and have noticed a positive difference in the health of my teeth.

If you don't have the option of buying natural toothpaste or remineralizing powder, you can make your own pretty easily. Here's how:

Homemade Tooth Powder Recipe

4 Tbsp bentonite clay

4 Tbsp calcium carbonate powder

1 tsp baking soda (leave this out if you have metal braces)

1 tsp fine sea salt

1 tsp ground cloves

10 drops peppermint essential oil (optional)

Instructions:

Mix all ingredients together in a bowl until combined. Transfer your mixture into an old, clean glass jar to store. When you're ready to brush your teeth, wet your toothbrush in the sink before dabbing it into the jar of powder and brushing like normal.

In addition to your teeth, don't overlook your gums either. To clean them, a regular wooden toothpick is better than nothing, but I also like to use massaging gum picks every night before brushing.

Before you get upset with me for using a disposable plastic product, I want you to know that I tried—I mean, I REALLY tried to find a reusable option. However, my teeth are too tightly pushed together for the bigger, sturdier, reusable options to work. So I use one of these over and over until it breaks before I grab a fresh one.

I also tried natural dental floss for years. They make biodegradable dental floss, and if it works for you, PLEASE use it. Unfortunately, I haven't been able to find one that can get through my super tight teeth, so I was forced to go back to using Glide floss. I recently started using a water dental flosser, and I love it! I can get the food bits out of my teeth between meals without having to do a complete brushing routine.

Do whatever you have to do to keep your gums and teeth healthy! If you're concerned about your teeth or bones becoming brittle with age, consider taking a stinging nettle tea or supplement daily. Stinging nettle is high in calcium and other nutrients that can improve bone health just as well as, if not better than, a multivitamin (Bhusal et al., 2022).

No matter what your daily routine is right now, I want to impress upon you the importance of incorporating the healthy oral habits we have gone over in this section. Improving your diet and your oral health alone can result in enormous changes in your body's overall condition. Starting now—no matter what you have or haven't done in the past—you can greatly improve your chances of having a healthy future, specifically concerning the health of your gums and teeth.

Your hygiene has a great impact on your overall health, well-being, and self-esteem. It also plays a critical role in the impression you have on the people you meet and interact with. If you are making sure to clean your hands, body, hair, teeth, and gums on a regular basis, that is all it takes to have good hygiene—simple and uncomplicated, isn't it?

Chapter 16: Childbirth, Babies, and Children

I chose not to get an epidural when I was in labor with either of my children. It hurt like hell, yes, but it was the kind of pain with an end in sight. Because I could feel what was happening in my body, I knew when it was getting close to the time I needed to push. Even still, a doctor still told me to get the epidural because doctors in hospitals think they know your body better than you do.

Trust me, YOU know your body better than anyone else in the universe does, whether you choose to pay attention to it or not. Hopefully by the time you've finished reading my book, you'll start paying more attention to your body and making decisions that are in line with what you know is right for you.

When you push a baby out vaginally, you are using the same muscles that you use to poop. When you start pushing when you're in labor, you poop—right there on the table in front of the doctors and nurses. It's completely normal and part of the process. Don't *ever* let anyone tell you otherwise or shame you for pooping while you're giving birth.

In fact, you're SUPPOSED to poop when giving birth vaginally. As the baby comes out, it touches some of the fecal leftovers and bacteria that came out with your poop. The bacteria or small poop remnants that get onto your baby as they are coming out serve to populate their microbiome and set it up for success

(Mueller et al., 2015). Because of this transfer of bacteria, your baby's body and digestive tract will eventually develop the ability to eat the same foods as you do.

This is why babies who are born via C-section often end up with more allergies, immune system problems, and gut issues than their vaginally born counterparts (Pantazi et al., 2023). Without being exposed to their mom's butt and crotch bacteria, their microbiome is lacking in that essential starter kit.

I breastfed both of my children for almost a year and a half each. If you can't breastfeed your children for any reason, there's no shame in that. However, if you have the capability to do so, I recommend it. Feeding your child breast milk for the first year of their life helps set them up with a healthy immune system for the rest of their life.

What follows are a few tips I learned firsthand from raising my kids that can probably help you (or another new mother) with your newborns/children.

Little Girls (children with a vagina or vulva like parts)

ALWAYS wipe poop from front to back! Not only does this make certain that no fecal matter accidentally gets pushed into the vulva, but it also gets the child used to the sensation so she knows what it feels like when she starts wiping her own bum. Make sure you remind her to do the same when she starts potty training.

This next part about little girls is going to make some people uncomfortable, but it is the truth and is a normal part of child development. Sometimes little girls masturbate. Essentially, she will self-stimulate with her hands or the surface of an object while lying face down on her bed for a period of time. When a toddler does this, they do not understand sex the same way adults do. They are simply exploring a part of their body they did not have regular access to before they graduated out of diapers. And yes, it feels good for them, and sometimes they may even orgasm. All the child knows is that what they're doing feels good; they do not understand the social implications of what they're doing.

I'm only going to say this once: Masturbation is a TOTALLY NORMAL part of human behavior! Although normal, it is important to teach your child that it is only meant to be done in private. As a parent, the best thing you can do if you see your child doing this at home is to either ignore the act or, if the child starts doing it on the sofa or at the dinner table, gently remind them that that is a private activity that should only be done in the privacy of their bedroom. If they begin doing it in public and are not old enough to verbally redirect, do your best to put their attention on something else so they stop (Weiss, 2021).

The first time you see this, you may be caught off guard; I know I was the first time I saw a little girl do this. Thankfully, I had Google and quickly figured out that child masturbation is a completely normal part of a child's development and self-exploration. For a more comprehensive look into this topic, I recommend Stephanie Amis' research paper, "Is This My Body? A Manual on Navigating Child Masturbation without Shame," which explores biological processes, historical contexts, and contemporary recommendations.

Following the previous instance, nobody yelled at the little girl, shamed her, or reacted negatively toward her in any way. I am very grateful that I was able to research what was happening and respond in an appropriate manner, without perpetuating fear and stigma of a formative and natural behavior done by most children. Respecting and accepting your child in this way is the first step toward *not* giving them a sexuality complex that they need therapy to address in years to come.

Speaking for myself, I felt sexually conflicted and repressed as I moved from childhood, through puberty, and into my early adulthood. I experienced incredible shame at doing anything sexual for a very long time, until after I hit puberty and grew breasts. During puberty, when my body started to change and develop, I became aware that almost all of my value as a woman was placed in the fact that I had large breasts and was capable of having babies. At the same time, I was made to feel that I was too masculine of a woman for any guy to like me other than for my ability to bear children.

Had I received more affirmation that I am valuable—not for what I can do, not because of how I look, and not based on how closely I adhere to definitions of "femininity"—I would have felt far more secure in myself as I moved through such developmental years of my life. As time has passed, we've thankfully become more willing and able to have these open and honest conversations as a collective. Parents, as your daughter moves through puberty, let her know that sex is not something she needs to fear or feel ashamed of.

Little Boys (children born with a penis or partial penis)

Circumcision has been and remains a hotly debated topic to this day, causing many new parents to struggle to make the age-old decision. A big part of the reason I chose to have my son circumcised was because his father was. I have known men who were circumcised, and I have known ones who were not. From experience, I learned that uncircumcised men are able to more easily contract certain infections and diseases due to the extra folds of skin that hold moisture and bacteria around the penis head. When personally faced with the decision after having my son, it was challenging, to say the least.

Circumcision removes the foreskin at the head of the penis (Earp, 2015). The removal of this protective layer of skin from the shaft introduces dryness and chafing on a very sensitive part of the body. This often poses issues during intercourse, as it is more difficult to maintain necessary lubrication. It also removes many of the nerves in the penis that are responsible for the sensation of pleasure during sex.

Knowing everything I know now, I do not recommend circumcision, as I think its drawbacks outweigh its benefits. I am not telling you what you should do concerning your child's body or that my logic is infallible; I am simply weighing in with the experience and knowledge that I have. Do what you think is best for your child with the information that you have. You have the advantage of being able to do your own research and read the personal accounts of others, allowing you to make a much more informed decision than parents were able to make before the internet was readily accessible and available to the average person.

Regardless of if your baby is circumcised or not, baby erections can happen. This is something that surprises a lot of new parents, but it is completely normal. Your son cannot control it when his little willy shoots straight up. This frequently coincides with the first time your son pees in your face. Keep your mouth closed when changing your baby boy in case this does occur. If it does happen and you're caught unawares with your mouth open, it may be a little gross, but you'll live.

In addition to experiencing occasional erections, young boys may masturbate or play with their penises. You may notice him doing so once he stops wearing diapers, as he will have gained access to a part of his body he did not have access to before. Again, this is a completely normal part of a child's development; they are simply exploring their anatomy and new sensations. When you see him doing this, just remind him to not do it in front of company, outdoors, or anyplace but the privacy of his own bedroom (Weiss, 2021).

As with little girls, it is important that you do not shame little boys for doing something that is a natural and formative part of their development. For further information on this topic, you can refer to Stephanie Amis' research paper, "Is This My Body? A Manual on Navigating Child Masturbation without Shame." While both little boys and little girls should be allowed to explore their anatomy without fear or stigmatization, it has been found that little boys benefit from firm redirection more than they do permissive parenting, especially in regard to sexual behavior (Kincaid et al., 2012). What is important is that you set your child up for success in their younger years so that they can then navigate puberty (and their sexuality) in a healthy way.

Finally, when your son starts taking baths or showers by himself, make sure he knows to wash his butthole. Teach him this from a very young age before there is embarrassment surrounding the topic (especially if you are a mother who is teaching your son). I shouldn't have to say this, but please assure your son that he is NOT gay for washing his butthole; it is simply a part of maintaining good hygiene. (And even if he decides he is gay someday, assure him that you'll love him anyway.) Don't raise a son who leaves skid marks everywhere he goes.

What follows are suggestions for both/all genders of babies and children. Here's what I've learned from years of experience being a mom:

Bath time

Give that baby a bath! Every 2-3 days should be more than sufficient for bathing an infant, except when they've had a blowout and are covered in poop. Then, by all means, bathe that kid!

Be mindful of the ingredients in soap marketed for infants. I fell for the "Johnson & Johnson Baby Shampoo" trap the same as most new parents do. Nowadays, if I had a baby, a good bar of unscented goat milk soap would be my go-to.

When your child gets a little older, this is a great trick to teach them during bathtime that will help them remember the most important areas to clean: **Wash your ABCs**—armpits, butt, and crotch. (You can thank my second husband's mom for that one.) As long as they have time to wash their ABCs, the rest of their body should be okay for a little while if a longer cleaning has to wait.

Private Parts

Make sure your child knows that **NO ONE** is allowed to touch their private parts without the child's permission. And if they feel uncomfortable in any way, they should say so and tell you about it as soon as possible. Obviously, you will need to help them wash and wipe down there when they are too young to do it for themself, and occasionally a doctor may need to take a look. Otherwise, that area is for your child and *them* alone.

I suggest you do not teach your child a cutesy name for their private parts. If you teach little Sarah that her vulva is called a "cookie," and one day she tells her teacher that Uncle Marty keeps trying to poke her cookie, the teacher is not going to understand or realize there is a problem. Crotch, pee-pee, wiener, whatever you call it, just make sure it's a word other adults will recognize.

Diaper Rash

When diaper rash happens, many parents go crazy with special creams trying to get rid of the problem. No medicine is too expensive to save our baby's bottom. However, diaper rash happens when moisture gets trapped next to the skin for long periods of time. Sure, you can rub calendula salve on it to soothe the rash, but a salve or cream is only going to trap the moisture against the skin for even longer.

What's the real cure for diaper rash? Set that baby's bum free!

Take their diaper off and allow your baby to be butt naked for a while. Let them lie on a towel or old blanket (something you don't mind them peeing or pooping on) while their skin airs out. This works best if you can do it outdoors in the sunshine (preferably in your backyard rather than an area where other people may walk by). If it's too cold outside, let your baby go bare buns on the kitchen floor for ten minutes or so—long enough for the moisture to evaporate from their sore bum.

You can spread a thin layer of calendula oil or salve over the red, angry parts of their skin if you think it will help them, but the rash will go away on its own after a few treatments of airing out their skin that is usually covered by a diaper, making sure that butt is completely air-dry.

(DO NOT use a hair dryer for this. They are too hot and will result in injury. I'm including this just in case someone is so desperate as to try this.)

Diapers

After a bath or a period of airing out, it's time to re-diaper. Please cloth diaper if you can. It's so much better for your baby and for the environment. Just as your body does better in breathable, natural fabrics, so does your baby's.

How do you wash cloth diapers? After scraping the solid waste off the diapers into the trash, give the cloth diapers a preliminary wash in the sink. Then, you can throw them in the washing machine to wash. Run a main hot wash with detergent to clean the diapers. Make sure to use a sensitive laundry detergent made with clean, simple ingredients that will not irritate your baby's skin. Do a final rinse so no detergent remains. Wring out your cloth diapers and hang them to dry (drying in the sun is best if possible). For more information on the subject, you can visit Green Mountain Diaper's web article, "Washing Diapers."

Pacifiers

If you're going to offer your baby a pacifier, consider getting an orthodontic one. I do not recommend allowing your child to walk around all day with a pacifier in their mouth. Prolonged use of a pacifier has been linked to late development of speech and vocabulary (Kanellopoulos & Costello, 2024). It can also cause their teeth to come in crooked. I recommend you save the pacifier for naptime or bedtime as an extra layer of comfort. Most children are emotionally ready to stop using a pacifier between 2 and 4 years old. Both of my kids stopped just before age 2. But they also had a boob in their mouth for long periods of time, so I'm pretty sure the silicone was far less appealing.

Teeth

Do not rub brandy or bourbon on your baby's gums to numb them when they start teething. The baby will get addicted to the flavor very quickly and will constantly cry for more, putting you in a worse position than you were in to start with. You'll have to cut them off like a belligerent drunk guy at happy hour.

You don't need to brush a baby's gums, but once they have a couple teeth popping through, you'll want to start brushing their teeth. They make baby toothbrushes that are little rubber nubs attached to a tube you place over your finger. Then rub some edible baby toothpaste onto their teeth with its help. You will want to find a toothpaste that is sugar-free. Again, I want to emphasize that once that baby gets teeth, those teeth need to be taken care of.

I have two children, a son and a daughter—I've been through it all. My daughter never wanted to brush her teeth when she was little, to the point that I recall holding her down and forcibly brushing them for her. Not my proudest parent moment, but at the time I felt it had to be done. My son didn't mind and certainly didn't want me holding him down, so he half-ass brushed his teeth every morning and night. I figured half-assed brushing was better than none at all.

Learning to Walk

If you decide to put shoes on your baby, especially if they're at the stage where they're starting to pull themselves up or begin walking, please make sure you put them in soft-soled shoes. These are like leather moccasins that offer just enough protection from the ground that they won't hurt themselves while also allowing their feet to make contact with the surface below them. Barefoot shoes for babies!

Humans developed the ability to walk before shoes were invented. Your feet cannot learn to walk properly in modern shoes. Starting your infant out in a set of trainers sets their feet up for disaster for the rest of their life. Barefoot or shoes that mimic being barefoot are best for your baby (and for you too). Barefoot shoes for babies (and adults) can be found online; I have included my favorites in the quick links section of this book to save you some time and searching.

Finally, skip buying your baby a walker of any kind. Walkers delay their development and learning to walk (Burrows & Griffiths, 2002). A walker allows the baby to lean on it for balance and push off the ground to roll the apparatus around rather than learning how to hold their own body up and control their center of gravity. They need to develop balance and core body strength in order to walk on their own. Putting them into a walker allows them to get around the house while also being lazy and not developing the proper skills they need to start walking. I had a balancing toy for my kids when they were babies. One of those bouncing harnesses that hangs in your doorway could also be great exercise for their little legs.

You want to allow your baby to crawl as long as they prefer! Don't force them to start walking just because you want them to. Babies develop their sense of spatial awareness while they are crawling around on the floor. It helps them develop motor coordination as well. If you allow your baby to crawl all over the place, they will develop a good sense of where and how to move their physical body through the world (in relation to everything else). They'll also develop a better sense of how far they can reach and how much space their body takes up in a room.

Allowing someone to develop at their own pace, whether they are a baby, your child, or someone whom you are mentoring in some way, is key to them developing the independence and confidence they need to succeed.

Now that we have covered the basics—healthful practices, preventative measures, and other helpful advice—it's time to delve into common afflictions, ailments, and remedies that can help reduce or eliminate them. While the remedies listed in the next part are generalized to be applicable to the majority of people, always do your own research or check with your doctor if you have a condition that is not addressed here.

For most of you, though, I think you'll be quite pleased to finally have a direct answer to the question "What do I do about [fill in the blank]?"

Now, let's answer it!

Part Two: Healing Remedies

Remedies to Aid Your Health—Your Siding

Do you remember how we talked about the foundation of your health being like the foundation your house is built on? Now, we are going to get into remedies, which serve as your siding—very helpful at stopping leaks and creating a protective barrier, but not the only thing you need to build a strong house.

How do I think like an herbalist?

Step one of thinking like an herbalist: When you or someone you know has a problem, ask, "What do you think is causing the problem?" Then ask yourself the following question: "What is causing the problem based on my knowledge and experience?"

You can't find the solution until you know what the problem is.

If a woman comes to you saying she has "tried everything" to stop her hair from falling out, what is the problem? If you answer that her hair is falling out, you're wrong. Hair loss is merely a ***symptom*** of a much larger problem. What could the problem be? That's where you want to focus your questions. What's your diet like? Have you had any recent blood tests done? Do you have hormonal imbalances? Are you anemic?

There are many questions an herbalist asks to get to the root cause of someone's problem. This book is not an exhaustive resource for all problems and all solutions. Instead, this book aims to get the gears in your brain turning in the same direction mine do when I am faced with a health-related problem.

There are no absolutes. Not every remedy or herb will help every person. Occasionally, someone may have a negative or opposite reaction to an herb than what I or another herbalist has described. If an herb you have been taking has not had any noticeable effect on you (or worse, has affected you in a negative way) after more than two weeks of taking it, I recommend you stop taking it and try again with a different herb.

There *are* some conditions you need a doctor to treat. Modern medicine can be miraculous when applied correctly. Sometimes herbs and food aren't going to be enough. Herbs can often help, but they aren't always the answer.

Play it safe with anyone you are helping. If a person is on any medications, look up whether their medication is going to interact with any herbs you think you want to recommend to them. I recommend you get a good herb/drug interaction book, like Francis Brinker's *Herbal Contraindications and Drug Interactions: Plus Herbal Adjuncts with Medicines, 4th Edition.* Of course, you can also use Google to do this as well.

If you (or the person you are assisting) are experiencing any alarming symptoms or want to stop taking a medication, it is important to speak with a doctor. *Occasionally*, you can replace someone's pharmaceutical prescription with a natural herbal equivalent (an herbal formula that has the same action in the body), but this is not always the case. Do not assume that you (or your client) will be able to stop taking all medications just because you started taking herbs. In some cases, simply implementing the nutritional protocol in this book will heal your symptoms. It all depends on the person and what actions they implement.

Thinking like an herbalist starts with the understanding that every human body is different. The herbal formulas I give you in this book are made with herbs that are generally considered to be safe. However, ANYONE can have an allergic reaction to ANYTHING. Please be cautious and start small if you're taking or giving an unfamiliar herb for the first time.

Before you start making your own herbal remedies, you'll want to acquire a decent herbal encyclopedia or The Modern Herbal Dispensatory. I refer to this book regularly because, even though it's not an exhaustive resource, it's a quick reference that has all the necessary information you need to craft great herbal medicines right in one book. It's important to craft your own library of resources whether you're a practicing herbalist or just want to take care of your own family's needs. My book should be part of your library, not your only resource on herbalism.

The following remedies and recipes I give you are based on treating a person who has no major medical conditions and is not on any pharmaceutical medications that could adversely interact with herbs. If a person is generally in good, stable health, these remedies and recipes can be tried at any time (after research, consideration, and consultation).

What you find here is not an exhaustive list of every ailment (or remedy) known to man. This is a general list of problems my family members or I have faced, as well as some problems I have helped clients with. What follows is my answer to "What would Amelia do if she had this symptom?" Please remember, I don't know everything!

One thing I DO know is that if you're the kind of person who gets sick frequently, you need to look deeper into the root cause of the problem. A weakened immune system or a really strong allergic reaction could be a sign of leaky gut or a nutritional deficiency.

Please use common sense! If you slice your finger down to the bone, don't just rub plantain on it and call it a day. Go to the hospital and get stitches! If you step on a rusty nail out in the goat pen, go to the doctor and get a tetanus shot. Sometimes a doctor or a hospital is necessary.

If it were my son or daughter, someone else I loved, or myself I was treating, this is exactly what I would do to solve each of these problems. As with everything else, please use your best judgment on the severity of your problem; if you think it's serious enough that you need to call a doctor, please do so. There is no shame in asking for help.

Chapter 17: Protecting Your Mental Health While Helping Others

Once people find out you're an herbalist, you'll likely be inundated with the question, "What herb can I take for this?"

Most people want you to throw herbs at them the same way a doctor throws pharmaceutical drug at them. They don't realize there is any difference. But you know better now. You want to help solve problems from a holistic approach, so you're going to ask them questions. And eventually, the solution may be more complicated than what they're willing to try.

It's okay to not help everyone who asks you for help. It's okay to say no if you are unable to assist them for any reason. It's okay if you try your hardest, but Grandma still refuses to listen to you and change her diet. Everyone has free will and experiences this lifetime to learn lessons.

You are learning that nature is a powerful healer and that our bodies are majestic symphonies that rely on a delicate balance of nutrition to make them function in harmony with our needs, wants, and desires. *Grandma* is learning that maybe she would live longer in her next lifetime if she wasn't such a stubborn pain in the ass.

You also need to be aware, if you're trying to help other people, that other people are not always going to be compliant with your suggestions. If you create an herbal formula for your cousin Joe that you know would make him feel better, but he never actually takes it, it doesn't matter how great the herbs are. Your formula isn't going to work.

From this point onward, I'm going to give you some remedies and recipes that I know and love and a very brief synopsis of the herbs I most commonly work with. I expect you to pick up an herbal encyclopedia and do more research about the plants discussed in this book on your own. I will also recommend books, teachers, and resources that I know and trust to have accurate information so that if I don't know the answer to something, I can point you toward someone who does.

The market is flooded with AI-generated books, blogs, and articles now, and I know how daunting it can be to figure out which sources to trust. There is a list of recommended reading at the end of the book for your convenience and use.

Remember how I said that every human body is different? Since we all have our own physical nuances, our bodies will each react slightly differently to each herb. For instance, mullein leaf tea can help someone deal with their dry, raspy cough and help move lymph through their body when they've been sick. Although rare, it's possible to come across a person who has either no reaction or even an adverse reaction to that same cup of mullein tea. It's important to start small with people who have not taken herbs medicinally before. (Use the same caution when helping a young child as well.)

Your body will tell you everything you need to know about your health. You just need to learn how to read it and talk with it. Learning to be in tune with your body is an indispensable life skill. Whether you're treating a chronic issue in yourself or someone else, you want to get to the root cause of the problem by understanding the person. If you *use* herbs the same way you would use a drug from the pharmacy, you're alleviating the symptoms for a while, but you aren't solving the actual problem. Let's change that!

Chapter 18: First-Aid Solutions and Preparation

Thankfully, I haven't had to use much in the way of first-aid solutions, but what I have are simple enough first-aid measures you can take for yourself, your kids, or whoever may need it, especially in a situation where your next step is a trip to the emergency room.

I do not have a ton of experience with first aid application. I'm not an EMT—I'm just an accident-prone woman with two kids who have hurt themselves more than a few times. The information in this chapter is VERY basic. If you want to learn more about herbal first aid, I have a couple resources I can direct you to:

7Song, an experienced herbalist, has written many informative blog articles on herbal first aid that you can find on his website. Additionally, The Holistic Herbalism Podcast recorded a great episode, titled "Herbs for First Aid and Disaster Response." (Both of these resources can be found in the Additional Resources section at the end of the book.)

If you have a gash or deep wound, you need to apply pressure right away. Wrap the wound with a piece of cloth or gauze if you can and apply pressure, holding the broken skin together until the bleeding stops. Get the bleeding person to the hospital as soon as possible for further medical attention.

Yarrow (*Achillea millefolium*) was used for centuries to help stop bleeding. However, it's not as good as hard pressure, a solid wrap, and a trip to the hospital. If you want to have a styptic powder on hand, I suggest you make one with dried, powdered yarrow leaves and flowers, dried usnea, and some cayenne powder.

For small cuts and scrapes, an herbal oil or salve made with calendula blossoms, plantain leaf, and self-heal is my go-to. I don't recommend you apply comfrey to an open wound, as comfrey tends to knit the skin together so quickly that it can trap bacteria inside the wound and put it at risk of infection.

Simple Healing Salve

2 Tbsp beeswax pellets

½ cup of infused oils (any combination of calendula oil, chamomile oil, plantain oil, self-heal oil, St. John's wort oil, and/or usnea oil)

20-30 drops of helichrysum essential oil

<u>Instructions</u>:

Add the beeswax and infused oils to a bowl or double boiler (I use a glass bowl set on top of a small pot half full of water) and heat until all the beeswax melts. Stir with a wooden or plastic utensil while heating. Then, add your helichrysum essential oil. Pour into tins or jars. Wait until your salve solidifies before putting the caps on and labeling them.

Always keep ice packs in your freezer in case of injury. Ice will help reduce inflammation and pain if someone has fallen and hurt themself or otherwise injured themself. A bag of frozen peas will serve the same purpose in a pinch. Additionally, try to find plastic-free bandages or gauze to stock your medicine cabinet and first-aid kit.

Comfrey is fantastic to have on hand (oil, salve, or fresh) in case someone sprains their ankle. A comfrey poultice or some strong comfrey-infused oil will help heal a bruise or a sprained wrist in just a few days. It can also be applied topically over a broken bone (after the bone has been set properly) to help reduce healing time. Alternatively, it can be taken as a daily tea for up to two weeks to help decrease the healing time of your broken bone.

While black walnut (*Juglans nigra*) extract is NOT the same thing as iodine, it DOES act very similarly. If you have the ability to make or buy a dropper bottle of black walnut tincture (made with the fresh green hulls of black walnuts and alcohol), you should keep that in your first-aid kit. It is a good second measure to clean a wound after you've rinsed it out with plain water first.

If you have accidentally allowed foreign matter or an infection to come into contact with the eye, make a strong tea with either chamomile flowers, rose petals, or both. Soak a cloth in the tea and apply it to the eye generously, with the intent that at least some of the liquid gets into the eye under the lashes. A person could also hold some of the cooled tea in their cupped hand and blink into the liquid, but using it as a compress is much easier. This is effective because rose tea and rose water are helpful and gentle anti-inflammatories.

This can be helpful in the case of pink eye (conjunctivitis), other types of eye infections, or if there is a shard of something in the eye. If you suspect someone has a shard or splinter in their eyeball, take them to the emergency room immediately! Only use this remedy in the event that you need to soothe them while they wait.

Again, I'm not a doctor or a surgeon. In the event of a serious medical emergency, please only use the tips I've given you here to help the person until they make it to a hospital.

Chapter 19: Constitution

Do you know your body's energetic constitution? Everyone has a different constitution—cold, warm, dry, damp, or some combination of these. As such, you need to take personal constitution into consideration when determining what herbs you take or recommend to someone else.

A man who frequently has pink cheeks and sweaty palms because he tends to run hot and damp should not be given cayenne pepper as a circulatory stimulant. It would only aggravate his already hot constitution. A woman who is always cold and has to repeatedly put hand lotion on because of how dry her skin is would probably not do well taking a remedy made with mint, hibiscus, or other highly cooling and drying herbs.

There are people who have spent the better part of their lives studying herbal energetics, so I want you to understand that the concept is far more nuanced than what I am describing in this book. In summation, **herbal energetics** refers to the action any given herb has on your body. Will it cool you down? Moisten dry skin? Make you feel warmer? Etc.

If you see an herb listed in a book next to the word "drying," does that mean it sucks the moisture out of your tissues (fleshy parts), does it tighten or pucker your tissues up, or does it cause your body to lose moisture (like a diuretic)?

There are many different ways in which an herb can exhibit one of these energetic qualities, so I suggest you research it more deeply.

Here are a few examples to get your mind working on this topic. Find and taste each herb, flower, fruit, root, and spice listed below if you can so you can experience the energetic effect it has on your body. (Fresh herbs, flowers, and roots if possible, but if dried, make a tea.) *Don't ingest witch hazel—apply it topically to feel its drying effect.*

Cooling herbs, flowers, and fruits: cleavers (*Galium aparine*), peppermint (*Mentha spp.*), self-heal (*Prunella vulgaris*), hibiscus (*Hibiscus rosa-sinensis*), cucumber (*Cucumis sativus*), and watermelon (*Citrullus lanatus*).

Warming herbs, root vegetables, and spices: ginger (*Zingiber officinale*), garlic (*Allium sativum*), cayenne (*Capsicum annuum*), cinnamon (*Cinnamomum verum*), and nutmeg (*Myristica fragrans*).

Drying herbs and flowers: lady's mantle (*Alchemilla vulgaris*), stinging nettle (*Urtica dioica*), witch hazel (*Hamamelis virginiana*), elderflower (*Sambucus nigra*), and rose (*Rosa rubiginosa*).

(Note: Most herbs are drying to the body in some capacity, so it's important that you balance out your formulas with a moistening herb, especially if the person you're helping has a particularly dry constitution.)

Moistening herbs and flowers: licorice root (*Glycyrrhiza glabra*), marshmallow (*Althaea officinalis*), slippery elm (*Ulmus rubra*), and evening primrose (*Oenothera biennis*).

Another concept I want to introduce you to is **synergy**. Every herb contains many different phytochemicals, also called constituents. There is synergy in each individual herb amongst its many constituents so that the herb works as one cohesive, whole medicine. But there is also a synergistic effect between the human body and the herb. An herb won't act the same in a laboratory Petri dish as it will work inside the human body. In other words, synergy is the interaction among a single herb's or multiple herbs' various constituents, which interact inside and in cooperation with the human body.

Multiple herbs combined together can often exhibit an even more complex and broad synergy—their individual constituents working together as a cohesive whole to accomplish their tasks alongside the synergy of the human body. Plant chemistry is a beautiful, choreographed dance of healing held inside our cells, and all we notice from the outside is whether we're finally feeling better.

This chapter merely scratches the surface of this concept. To dive deep into the topic of herbal energetics, I recommend *Energetic Herbalism* by Kat Maier. And to learn more about plant chemistry, I recommend studying with Lisa Ganora at her school, Herbal Constituents.

In addition to studying concepts such as constitution and synergy, it is paramount you get to know the PERSON you are trying to help rather than just throwing herbal remedies at their SYMPTOMS. If you would like specialized support for your own body, you can contact me about a one-on-one consultation.

Chapter 20: Pain and Inflammation

"Pain" is a word that can mean SO many things! Are you in pain physically, mentally, emotionally, sexually, or spiritually? For the scope of this chapter, I'm only going to write about ways to treat physical pain.

Pain is the sensation you register in your brain when some part of your body is inflamed. You're feeling the pain because the inflamed tissue is pressing against a nerve. Inflammation is actually your body trying to heal itself.

There are two types of inflammation: acute and chronic. **Acute inflammation** is what happens after you've been injured or suddenly gotten sick. For example, if you contract strep throat, the back of your throat may swell up with inflammation while your body attempts to heal itself. Or if you fall and hurt your leg, it will often swell and bruise, indicating inflammation. Acute inflammation can last from a few days up to a few weeks, depending on the condition.

Chronic inflammation occurs when your body continues sending the inflammatory response to a certain area despite the danger posed by the initial injury having passed. Basically, your body is continuing to receive the pain response even though the reason it started is long over.

Many people run to the pharmacy and buy ibuprofen, acetaminophen, or aspirin. Sometimes they are even prescribed high-powered painkillers like OxyContin or morphine. These medications are NOT meant to be taken long-term and can, in fact, be harmful (or even addictive in the case of opiates). Most commonly, they can cause you to develop a stomach ulcer with continued use. I suggest you keep a small amount in your medicine cabinet in case of emergencies, but take herbal remedies whenever possible.

Acute inflammation, while unpleasant, can be addressed with various pain-relieving herbs such as birch bark, meadowsweet, wild lettuce, or willow bark. I make a tincture or an infused oil with these herbs (preferably fresh when possible) to extract their pain-relieving components. There are other pain-relieving herbs, such as devil's claw and kratom, but I prefer to recommend herbs that I personally work with and know do the job.

(A warning about kratom: I have heard of this being the only viable replacement for opiates, but kratom is no less addictive than opium. It is my recommendation that you avoid these two altogether once you wean yourself off of them.)

While you can experience temporary relief from chronic pain using the aforementioned pain-relieving herbs, it isn't a permanent fix. You're not resolving the problem by throwing painkillers at it—natural or not. Now you're saying, "But how do I solve my pain permanently?!" I hear you.

You need to understand that your emotions can and do cause physical pain. Have you ever been upset over something and then had a stomachache? Of course; all of us have. That's your proof that emotions affect your body for better or worse. If you regularly experience emotional pain (ranging from mild to severe), it is going to affect your body. If this is the position, you're in, all the herbs are going to do is act as a pain tranquilizer, not a healer. (If you're being abused in any way, shape, or form—

physically, mentally, or emotionally—please seek qualified professional help.)

Following the dietary protocol outlined at the beginning of this book and making small lifestyle changes, such as going on walks or exercising outdoors as often as possible, will immensely help toward alleviating your chronic pain. However, as mentioned previously, every human body is different. You may be best served by having a consultation with an experienced herbalist or naturopath who can address your specific concerns and give you personalized suggestions.

If I've been in pain for more than a couple weeks, I try to figure out what's causing it. Did I twist my back lifting the heavy garage door again? Did I sleep in a certain position that made my leg cramp? Deciphering the CAUSE of your chronic pain is the first step toward finding a viable solution to treat it, whether that's through diet, exercise, therapy, supplementation, etc.

Understanding WHY you hurt where you hurt is critical. Most people with back pain don't realize that it's not their back causing the pain. It's their glutes, hamstrings, psoas, and other muscles pulling on the muscles in their hips and back. *Back pain can also be caused by a herniated disc, which needs to be diagnosed by a doctor. However, don't jump to a spinal injury as the cause unless you have reason to believe that may be the case. *

I recently saw a ROLFING specialist (Rob Martin of Rolf Bodyworks in Sterling, CT) who helped ease my pain greatly. ROLFING (also known as Structural Integration) is a method of realigning your body's muscles, tendons, and connective tissues back to where they are anatomically meant to be (Dr. Ida Rolf Institute, 2019).

The ROLFING specialist I saw told me that the muscles attached to my tailbone were frozen, causing my hips to be held in an offset position. Carrying my weight like this every day resulted in pain and stiffness over time. I have tight psoas muscles on both sides of my body, and my hip flexors are also tight and weak. Additionally, my hamstrings are tight from sitting far too often (working at my desk) instead of exercising and moving around. This was causing me to feel an immense amount of pain in my lower back region until I started exercising those muscle groups to strengthen them. Fascia flossing—stretching and breaking up the connective tissue between the muscle layers in your body—is a fantastic daily practice that can reduce your pain as well (Johns Hopkins Medicine, n.d.).

Eating a diet that reduces your inflammatory load is critical to managing chronic pain. Simply avoiding highly processed foods like bologna, cakes, cookies, crackers, pepperoni, soda, and other prepackaged foods should help ease inflammation-related conditions. Studies have proven that diets that are high in sugar and processed foods increase overall inflammation (Ma et al., 2022). Although my diet is about as anti-inflammatory as it gets, I still need help from regular stretching, massage, and seeing a ROLFING specialist whenever I can to realign my muscles. Never discount the help you can receive from seeing an experienced chiropractor or deep tissue massage therapist.

Having covered the difference between acute and chronic pain and lifestyle-based measures you can take to counteract inflammation, here are the herbs I rely on most often to treat inflammation:

I take **turmeric** (*Curcuma longa*) twice a day on days when my pain is particularly bad. For years, turmeric has been known as a powerful anti-inflammatory. However, it doesn't work well for some people, in which case you may want to experiment with other anti-inflammatory herbs like cayenne and ginger.

When supplementing turmeric, you must be sure that your supplement combines turmeric with piperine (black pepper), as the combination of these two herbs increases turmeric's inflammation-modulating effects. The combination also reduces the chance of the curcuminoids in turmeric escaping your body through natural channels of elimination (such as through the liver) before they have a chance to combat inflammation and pain.

Please note: Turmeric is NOT curcumin. Curcumin is the main healing constituent of turmeric. Black pepper is NOT piperine. Piperine is the main healing constituent of black pepper. Herbs are whole medicines in themselves, full of dozens of different constituents that all work with one another synergistically. Oftentimes, they have an even stronger effect on the human body when combined with other herbs. This is part of the concept of synergy.

I also like making my own golden milk with some turmeric, black pepper, ginger root, cloves, and cardamom. To see how I make mine, you can watch my golden milk tutorial video (linked in the Additional Resources section at the end of the book).

Goldenrod (*Solidago spp.*) is an inflammation-modulating herb, which means that it can help reduce the inflammation your body is feeling when taken daily over time. The best way to experience goldenrod's pain-relieving power is as an herbal-infused oil (Bennett, 2013). I also love working with goldenrod as a tea or tincture to help reduce my allergic load in the springtime.

Another herb that works great as an infused oil when applied topically is **cayenne pepper** (*Capsicum annuum*). Cayenne can be made into an infused oil, and when you apply it, not only does it help relieve your pain, it also warms the area and increases circulation. This can be especially helpful for rheumatism—the pain a person experiences from feeling too cold when they have damaged nerves.

My two favorite pain-relieving plants are black birch and wild lettuce. The only thing you need to understand about these herbs is that while they are FANTASTIC at reducing the pain you are feeling (their effects last several hours), they are not going to stop the CAUSE of your pain.

Black birch (*Betula lenta*) contains methyl salicylates, which act in the body very similarly to aspirin. They're like a minty version of the same compound that's found in willow bark. (I prefer the flavor of birch over willow, and it's much easier to identify in my opinion.)

Another plant that contains this compound is **wintergreen** (*Gaultheria procumbens*), though it's much harder to find and forage a large enough amount of this small evergreen groundcover plant than it is to harvest black birch bark. (Note: do not give birch to dogs, as it contains natural xylitol, which is toxic to them.)

Wild lettuce (*Lactuca virosa*) is the kind of pain reliever I will take if I've been out hiking or working in the garden all day and I strained my back, if I fell in a hole and hurt my leg, or if I ever broke a bone. It is one of the strongest painkillers you can find and forage in nature. It is not as strong as opium, but it is the best when it comes to dealing with a major injury naturally. To learn more about wild lettuce, you can watch my short video lesson (linked in the Additional Resources section at the end of the book).

As with all herbs and supplements that are new to you, it's generally recommended you start with a smaller dose and work your way up. Dosage is dependent on the herb you're taking, your size and weight, your tolerance to certain constituents (and alcohol if taking a tincture), and other factors that are specific to you. While there are other herbs known to help relieve pain, the ones detailed in this chapter are the ones I work with most. (That herbal encyclopedia you're buying is going to be mighty handy when you start looking for pain-relieving plants that grow near you!)

Getting up and moving your body around as often as you can, paying attention to the flow of lymph through your body (because stagnant lymph can cause pain too), and maintaining a low-inflammation diet are your keys to reducing your chronic pain. But knowing WHERE and WHY you hurt helps most of all.

Chapter 21: Boosting Your Immune System

For those of you who are looking to add another layer of prevention on top of a balanced diet, there are some herbs you can keep on hand or take daily that will give your body an edge over the viral enemies of the world. Additionally, fire cider, garlic, medicinal mushrooms, and probiotics can boost your immunity, whether you are currently healthy or sick.

70-80% of your immune cells reside in your gut (Wiertsema et al., 2021), which is one of the many reasons I keep drilling home the importance of gut health. When your gut is in disarray, it is likely your immune system is too (since they're so interconnected). Alternatively, when you feed your body immunity boosters, you're left with a happy gut and strong immune system.

Here are further descriptions of my favorite immunity boosters:

Echinacea (*Echinacea purpurea*): Since the 90s, Echinacea has been touted as a miracle herb for helping people get over the common cold (Zhai et al., 2007). Whether you're taking the root or the flower, it is like giving your body's "regular" gas tank a big bottle of moonshine. It is NOT something to be taken every day as an immunity tonic, and if you are on immunosuppressant drugs, it would be best to avoid this plant altogether. For everyone else, keep a bottle of Echinacea root tincture, and take 2 droppers full every day while you are sick (with a virus). Don't take it for longer than two weeks consecutively.

Elderflower (*Sambucus nigra*): Believe it or not, tincture form is best for taking this herb. The tea will work, but the lovely smell of fresh elderflowers quickly turns to a dirt flavor in your teacup. I will take 1-2 droppers full of elderflower tincture at the onset of cold or flu symptoms. (Note: ElderFLOWER is best at the onset of a virus, while elderBERRY is what I would suggest you take if you already have a virus and are trying to get over it.)

Fermented foods: I'm happy to be finding more companies making fermented foods that you can purchase from the store, such as kimchi, fermented pickles, and even fermented seaweed (my favorite). Fermented foods increase the diversity of your gut microbiome and decrease the amount of inflammatory proteins found in the digestive tract, effectively reducing your chances of developing type 2 diabetes or rheumatoid arthritis (Weaver, 2021).

Fire cider: This can be used as a preventative or a cure. The preventive dose is about 1 tbsp daily. If you are sick, 1 full shot glass worth will help kill what ails you. (You can find my recipe in Chapter Twenty-Three.)

Garlic (*Allium sativum*): Yep, the stuff you buy at the grocery store works just fine. If I feel a cold or virus coming on, I'll eat a raw clove of garlic. It burns a little going down and gives me garlic breath for a couple of hours, but I have had success doing this on multiple occasions and cutting off the cold before it had time to take hold. It also helps your body fight off microorganisms. Eating garlic at dinner every night is a must in my household for its many health benefits.

Medicinal mushrooms: Reishi (*Ganoderma tsugae*) is my favorite immunity booster, followed closely by chaga (*Inonotus obliquus*), maitake (*Grifola frondosa*), and turkey tail (*Trametes versicolor*).

Mushroom extracts build up in your system over time, so you should be taking a double-extracted tincture of the mushroom fruiting body daily to see real benefits from any of these. Here, "double-extracted" means that the mushroom constituents were extracted in both alcohol and water. Alcohol extracts the triterpenes, while water extracts the beta-glucans (Hutchison, 2021). I am a huge proponent of taking medicinal mushrooms!

Probiotics: DO NOT underestimate the power of gut health when it comes to preventing sickness! I would caution you against eating yogurt or kefir when you're sick since the dairy may cause more mucus to build up at the back of your throat. I recommend taking 1-2 capsules of a probiotic daily. My favorite probiotic is Silver Fern™ Ultimate Probiotic.

While the previously listed immunity boosters are great at what they do, vitamin C (Carr & Maggini, 2017) and zinc (Shankar & Prasad, 1998) are *crucial* to maintaining a strong, healthy immune system. You should be getting vitamin C and zinc in your diet if you're eating plenty of fresh or dried fruits and meat or seafood. The forager in me will be super happy if I catch you eating (or drinking) rose hips for their vitamin C, and a can of smoked oysters can shoot your zinc levels through the roof (in a good way). Although these two stand out, it is important that you're getting ALL your daily nutritional needs met to support overall immune function.

There's a difference between utilizing the power of herbs to "boost" your immune system during an acute bout of sickness and relying on herbs to run your immune system in place of taking care of your body. Your first line of defense should always be eating nutritious foods, drinking lots of water, and taking a walk every day. It really *is* that simple to support your health.

Chapter 22: Your Lymphatic System

Do NOT underestimate your lymphatic system when you are sick! And don't neglect it when you're well. Being conscious of habits that could cause lymph fluid to stagnate in your body is important. That can be as simple as remembering to get up and move around every hour, even on days you're stuck at the office or feeling like a couch potato and watching Netflix.

Your lymphatic system is a group of organs, tissues, and vessels that protect you from infection and keep a healthy balance of fluids moving throughout your body (Piedmont, n.d.). Your lymphatic system is comprised of your adenoids, bone marrow, lymph channels, lymph nodes, spleen, thymus gland, and tonsils (UnityPoint Health, n.d.). Swollen lymph nodes are a sign of common infections, like strep throat, but also more serious diseases like cancer.

Think of your lymphatic system as the garbage truck running around picking up the daily trash from all your other organ systems. If you don't empty out the truck once in awhile, things are going to get backed up and start to stink and decay real fast.

If you start feeling pain or swollen areas under your chin, in your neck area, in your armpits, under your clavicle, or in your groin, these are all signs of clogged lymph ducts. Your lymphatic system is basically like the Garbage Dump Highway inside your body. It runs from the crown of your head down to your feet, sucking up all the dead tissues, blood cells, viruses, and other junk that your body needs to get rid of. Your lymphatic system then transports all the matter that needs to be disposed of to your liver, skin, and urinary tract to be removed from your body.

The most important thing to remember is this: Your lymphatic system does not have a pump. Unlike your heart, which pumps blood throughout your body whether you're awake, asleep, drunk, sober, or falling from the sky in a parachute, your lymphatic system can only move stagnant lymph fluid through your body through MOVEMENT.

When you're sick, tired, feeling like crap, and hurting everywhere, the best thing you can do is get up off your butt and go take a walk outside. No, I don't care if it's cold out there. Get some clean, fresh air into your lungs and move your body! Even if you just stand outside your back door in your pajamas and snow boots, wiggling your arms in the air and jumping up and down like a clown with a frog down his shirt, as long as you're moving, you are helping to get that garbage highway rolling.

I bought a rebounder (mini trampoline) last winter, and it gets used nearly every day all year long, partly because I want to move lymph through my body and partly because it's fun as hell to jump on a trampoline. Just two or three minutes of jumping every day can have a powerful effect on your lymphatic drainage. I highly recommend it!

If you get sick in the dead of winter, your first inclination is likely to be to curl up on the sofa with some chicken soup, a blanket, and a movie. While this may feel more comfortable, it will actually make your virus quite cozy too. The best thing you can do is get dressed nice and warm and take yourself out for a short hike or walk, preferably in clean, fresh air. Your nose might run, but not only will the cool air help clear your sinuses, the physical movement will help push the virus out of your system and get you over the sickness even faster! I promise you will be the one laughing when you feel better in just a day or two when your partner (who refused to get out of bed when they were sick) is still sick with the same thing a week later.

Here are a few herbs you can rely on to support your lymphatic system in case you end up bedridden:

- Burdock root (*Arctium lappa*)
- Calendula (*Calendula officinalis*)
- Cleavers (*Gallium aparine*)
- Poke root (*Phytolacca americana*): *__Use caution!__ You need to make a tincture with this herb; the max dosage is 8 drops at a time, 2 times per day. More than that can cause violent vomiting or possibly death. I take 6 drops a day in the morning and it helps me with lymph issues. Do further research on this herb before you try it!*
- Red root (*Ceanothus americanus*)
- Stinging nettle (*Urtica dioica*): This is the one herb I would suggest you ALWAYS keep on hand in your apothecary, as it can be used to treat a wide variety of ailments. It's highly nutritious, somewhat drying, and can help reduce your body's allergic load. When in doubt, take nettles!
- Violet (*Viola spp.*): Both the leaf and flower are great at both cleansing lymph and soothing your throat, so a good herb to have on hand when you're sick

Remember how I said your lymphatic system doesn't have a pump? Making sure you get movement every day will help move the stagnant lymph through your body. It's better to send the garbage truck on to the dump as often as possible rather than allowing the full trucks to just sit in a parking lot rotting in the hot sun for days. Keep your metaphorical dump trucks (lymphatic system) moving regularly, and you'll have a fresh start to all your cellular processes to begin each new day.

Chapter 23: When You Do Get Sick—Common Infections and How to Treat Them

Despite all your best efforts, there will be times when you get sick. If not yourself, it may be your spouse, child, or household member who falls ill and needs to be taken care of. No matter who is sick, preventative measures remain important, namely frequent hand washing, taking immunity boosters, and maintaining lymphatic flow.

My protocol for a virus is the same whether the symptoms are sore throat, sneezing, stomach pain, or any other number of symptoms. However, various measures can be taken depending on whether you have just started feeling unwell or if you are in the full-blown thick of the virus. These suggestions are for both children and adults, with the caveat that a child may, of course, need a smaller dose of whatever remedy you're employing (based on their size).

The herbs and recipes in this section can help you recover from just about any viral infection, surgery, or sickness. However, if you begin experiencing symptoms you feel unequipped to handle at home or if your symptoms worsen, please go to the doctor for treatment.

The Common Cold (or whatever virus your kid brought home from school)

Whether it be the common cold or a different run-of-the-mill virus, I prioritize boosting the good bacteria in the gut to fight off the infection. In my experience, the best basic care you can implement when you feel yourself getting sick is going to the store and buying a bottle of **kombucha**. Any flavor will do, but I prefer the lemon/ginger combination when I get sick. Drink this slowly over the next several hours to boost your gut flora. You can also take a good-quality probiotic, but I find the bubbly, flavored kombucha to be both relaxing and soothing to an upset stomach.

I once worked as a delivery driver at a place where everyone had been getting sick with the flu and calling out sick. I thought I'd be fine until my turn came around. Thankfully, I was delivering to a bunch of health food stores at the time. Once the wave of fever and faintness started to hit me, I bought a bottle of kombucha and started sipping on it the rest of my route. Three hours later, I'd gone from feverish and lightheaded to perfectly fine.

My second suggestion provides equal parts comfort and nourishment: Make some **homemade bone broth**. Use some leftover chicken or buy a small pack of chicken from the store (you only need one chicken leg for this to work). Most grocery stores sell bones with very little meat or just some marrow visible. These are good to use, but the best bones to use are ones that come from a local small farm, so buy those if you can.

The vegetables may take a little more preparation. Any time I cook dinner, I save the little bits and scraps of celery ends, garlic nubs, onion ends, potato peels, etc., and put them in a Ziploc bag before sticking them in the freezer. I add to the bag every time I cook, and eventually, there's enough to make my bone broth recipe. If I roast a chicken and have picked off all the meat I can, I throw that into the big crock pot with my bag of veggie scraps, along with some salt and pepper. Then, I cook it on low for a day or so.

You can either drink your broth in a mug, use it as a base for soups, cook your rice and pasta in it, freeze it in batches for later use, or whatever else you can think of. You will get the most immune system benefits by drinking some of this warmed up every day, especially while you're sick. Bone broth is extremely helpful in healing the gut lining (Matar et al., 2025) and is my first go-to remedy for treating gut ailments.

Bone Broth Recipe

1-2 pounds of bones from pasture-raised animals (beef, chicken, lamb, and venison are best in my opinion, but any bones will work)

Tip: You can use a whole piece of meat with skin and fat to make a richer broth which will result in a higher fat content

Vegetable scraps (saved veggie ends, peels, and chunks from previous meal preparation, stored in a quart-size Ziploc bag in the freezer until ready for use)

If you don't have veggie scraps, use:

1 carrot, broken in half

1 onion, sliced into quarters (do not peel)

1 small potato, cut into chunks

1-2 celery sticks, chopped or broken small enough to fit in the pot

2 cloves of garlic, cut in half

Herbs and spices (astragalus root, black pepper, cinnamon, oregano, parsley, thyme, etc.—herbs and spices are based on your personal preference)

Optional: dried mushrooms (a handful will do)

Instructions:

Roast the bones at 350°F for half an hour with some salt and pepper (doing this step first helps produce a nice flavor, but isn't absolutely necessary).

Put your saved veggie scraps into your crock pot. Salt and pepper to your taste. I also like to add a little seaweed and some mushrooms if I have them, as well as whatever herbs or green things I can forage from the yard.

If you haven't been saving your veggie scraps, prepare your vegetables (don't bother peeling anything). Rough chop a carrot, a potato, and some celery (breaking them in half first). Cut an onion into quarters. Throw in those nasty little pieces of garlic that are hell to peel or two big cloves cut in half (you don't need to peel them). Then, follow the above step, adding your seasoning and any additions you wish to include.

Put your roasted bones in the crock pot with your vegetables; cover with water almost to the top. DON'T FORGET to add 1/4 cup of apple cider vinegar, which helps leach the minerals from the bones. Cook on low for 24 hours or more. The end result may need some extra salt (since it tends to cook off).

After it's finished cooking, strain the solids out with a colander and either pour a cup of the broth into a mug to drink (salt to your taste) or save (and freeze) it for later use. Toss the solids into your compost (or feed them to your chickens if you have that option).

Please note: if you have histamine intolerance you will want to make this recipe as stock instead. To do so, simply omit the cider vinegar and cook in a large pot for 2-3 hours rather than 24 hours.

Lastly, **fire cider** can help knock sickness out quick! Yes, you can buy some at the grocery store now, but it's wimpy compared to what you can make at home. A shot of my fire cider will put some hair on your chest and burn whatever ails you right out.

Dosage: Take ½ shot glass of this for an immune booster if you're starting to feel sick. If you are already sick or in the thick of a virus, take a whole shot. You can add some honey to it for taste, but I just knock it back like a sailor drinking hard rum on a cold night. It is not pleasant going down, but it will kill your cold in about 3 doses max.

I've been making this for so long that I improvise with my recipe, adding whatever ingredients I have available. Feel free to add or subtract a little here and there on the quantities. If you cannot find fresh ginger or turmeric, substitute 1 tbsp of each dried. You can follow the below recipe or follow along with my video tutorial (linked in the Additional Resources section at the end of the book).

Fire Cider Recipe

1-2 big, fat roots of fresh horseradish

2 thumbs of fresh ginger

2-3 thumbs of fresh turmeric

4 stalks of rosemary (~2 Tbsp)

2 Tbsp fresh thyme

2 lemons

3 bulbs' worth of garlic

2-3 yellow onions

2 hot peppers (whatever kind you have available)

2 liters raw apple cider vinegar

Instructions:

First, grate your horseradish into a big bowl (I use a bell grater and do this by hand).

Be very careful, as you are likely to skin your knuckles and bleed all over the place the first time you try this. But no amount of chopping compares to actually grating the fresh horseradish. Your eyes are going to water, your nose is going to run, and you won't be able to see through the horseradish tears. If you have goggles or something equivalent, try using those to shield your eyes. Otherwise, keep a paper towel nearby to blow your nose and plan on washing your hands frequently. Maybe try doing this outside. Although troublesome, it's totally worth it!

Mix all your herbs, fruits, and vegetables together in a big bowl, and then stuff them into a gallon or two half-gallon-sized jars. Pour the raw apple cider vinegar over your ingredients. If you still have airspace in the jar, you can top it off with regular 5% ACV to save some money.

Cover the jar with a plastic lid or line your metal lid with plastic wrap, as the apple cider vinegar will corrode a metal top. Allow this to sit in a dark place, shaking the jar occasionally, for at least

6-8 weeks. Then, strain the solids out, and store the liquid in a clean glass bottle.

Stomach Viruses

In the event you come down with a stomach virus, I would follow the same protocol I have laid out for treating the common cold. It's important to remember, though, whether it's a stomach bug or food poisoning: If you are experiencing diarrhea, it is best to let it run its course. Don't jump to your herb shelf and search for blackberry leaf or another astringent to stop the diarrhea. Allow your body to cleanse your system of whatever has offended it.

Herbs that help stop diarrhea should only be considered if the diarrhea is a chronic problem or has been going on for several days, as the body is clearly not absorbing any of the nutrition or fluids you're giving it. In the case of prolonged symptoms, you will want to consult a doctor about the problem as well, in case any medical tests are necessary.

Vomiting or Nausea

There are several instances when you may experience an upset stomach. You may be suffering the effects of food poisoning, morning sickness, motion sickness, a stomach virus, or stress. If you're a pregnant woman, you need to use caution with the amount of herbs you take for your nausea (don't take more than 2-3 cups of tea a day). The herbs used to treat nausea are the same for anyone dealing with regular, viral-induced nausea.

Please note that if you're experiencing nausea or vomiting due to an acute bout of food poisoning, it is best to let your body rid itself of what has caused the vomiting (the same as with diarrhea). Make yourself comfortable, hugging the toilet, and allow your body to expel the offending food/bacteria so it can get back to healing. You can decide what herbs to take after it's all out of your system.

My top 3 herbs for nausea:

- Ginger (*Zingiber officinale*)—fresh ginger grated into a cup with a small slice of lemon makes an excellent stomach-soothing tea.
- Peach leaf (*Prunus persica*)—can be taken as a tea or tincture, excellent for pregnancy-related nausea and motion sickness.
- Peppermint or spearmint (*Mentha spp.*)—best taken as a tea, but a tincture will do if it's all you have.

Strep Throat

To preface, I'm going to tell you a quick story: Back in 2015, I was a substitute teacher for several months. I got sick a LOT during that time. On one occasion, my throat began to hurt on one side every time I swallowed. I went to the doctor, and they tested me for strep throat. Sure enough, that's what I had. I was given a course of antibiotics and sent on my way.

Everything cleared up, and I was fine for about two weeks. Then it came back—same spot, same pain. I saw the doctor again and was given another course of antibiotics. It solved the strep for about a week and a half; then it was back again.

I learned my lesson this time. I did a little research online and decided to try a natural solution. I poured raw apple cider vinegar into a cup and gargled it in the back of my throat. It burned like hell! I would gargle and spit, gargle and spit, then gargle a tiny amount and swallow it. (At first it was kind of strong, so I diluted it with a little water, but I quickly built up a tolerance.) I gargled with ACV three times a day for two days. By the end of the third day, the pain was gone, and so was the strep. It never came back.

A year or so ago I told that story to my primary care doctor, and her eyes grew wide like saucers. She said, "Well… I guess that *would* work."

If you are dealing with strep throat (which usually feels like a sharp pain on one side of the back of your throat every time you swallow), simply pour some **raw apple cider vinegar** into a small glass or shot glass, water it down just a little (if you need to), and then use it to gargle at the back of your throat a few times. The last sip should be swallowed rather than gargled. Do this 2-3 times each day until the strep/pain clears.

Heavy Mucus or Tinnitus

I just want to note here, since we've been talking about sinus issues and being sick, that my go-to remedy for a sinus infection—tons of gunky mucus in the throat or sinuses—AND tinnitus (ringing in the ears) is the same: ground ivy (Swift, 2017).

Ground ivy (*Glechoma hederacea*) can be taken as a tea (1 tbsp dried to 8 oz hot water) 3-4 times a day or as a tincture 5 times a day (spaced out and taken over the course of the day). It's better than Mucinex for treating excess mucus, making it a staple in my allergy relief blends. It is a wild edible with a spicy, pungent flavor. And bonus: It's basically a weed, so you shouldn't have any trouble finding someone who will gladly let you pick some from their yard or garden.

Why have I mentioned tinnitus alongside heavy mucus? Well, in some cases, taking ground ivy can actually reduce or resolve tinnitus if it is caused by a buildup of fluid in the inner ear. Even if it doesn't stop your tinnitus, it is a very safe remedy to try, and at the very least, it will probably clear your sinuses out for a while.

Herbs for Coughing, Sneezing, and Mucus

You can work with the following herbs as a tea or a tincture; it's up to you. These are the herbs I reach for most often when I'm feeling unwell. When I'm sick, I prefer to drink herbal teas, as they help soothe my throat and mucous membranes. I'll provide a couple of tea recipes after I list the herbs.

The herbs are as follows:

- Bee balm (*Monarda fistulosa*): spicy, aromatic, and excellent in a blend to help cleanse the sinuses.
- Birch bark (*Betula lenta*): a little added to tea helps ease stomach pain if you're treating a stomach flu (keep away from dogs).
- Ginger (*Zingiber officinale*): a warming digestive herb that helps relieve stomachache.
- Ground ivy (*Glechoma hederacea*): great for expelling mucus.
- Juniper/Eastern red cedar (*Juniperus virginiana*): can be added along with a combination of thyme, sage, and oregano to an herbal sinus steam.
- Mullein (*Verbascum thapsus*): antispasmodic, lymphatic cleanser, and mucilaginous.
- Oregano (*Origanum vulgare*): Oil of oregano, made by infusing olive oil with dried oregano, can be indispensable in the case of an internal bacterial infection. It is also high in volatile oils and lends itself well to an herbal steam.

- Thyme (*Thymus vulgaris*): antiviral and antibacterial—kicks the common cold's butt.
- Yarrow (*Achillea millefolium*): acts as a natural febrifuge (helps reduce a fever or the pain that accompanies a fever).

I would additionally recommend garlic, lemon, and raw honey as remedies for coughing, sneezing, and mucus. Garlic (*Allium sativa*) helps boost your immune system by lowering inflammation and enhancing immune cell activity, as well as reducing the time you are sick with a cold or flu (Ansary et al., 2020). Whether it's cooked as part of your meals, infused in honey and taken medicinally, or eaten raw, garlic is an immunity-boosting superfood. In my book, garlic is medicine.

Lemon (*Citrus limon*) is high in vitamin C and soothing when used as part of an herbal blend. You can use the whole lemon, juice, or peel. Raw honey is anti-inflammatory and adds antioxidants along with a healthy dose of carbohydrates to your tea. Plus, it makes everything taste good. *Remember, don't give honey to infants under 1 year old. *

Tea has been taken medicinally for longer than history has been recorded (Huda et al., 2024). It's not hard to find a plant that smells nice, crush some up, put it into a cup, and pour water over it. That's really all there is to making a cup of tea at the most basic level.

I drink a cup of Earl Grey tea every morning at breakfast time and have done so since I was 12 years old, mostly because Captain Jean-Luc Picard of the USS Enterprise told me it was a good idea. I'm an Earl Grey fan and have tried many varieties. It's my comfort tea. I know that may sound funny to some, but it's not far off. Black tea contains L-theanine, a compound that helps relax your body and lower stress. It's no wonder the English demand a cup of tea during a stressful situation; I do too!

Herbal teas can be simple or complicated, medicinal or fun. They may contain one single herb or plant, or they may contain dozens (like some of the formulas used in Chinese medicine). I prefer to keep my teas around seven ingredients or less, both for ease of formulation and because it's easier to remember a simpler formula.

Formulating herbal blends is both an art and a science, and I encourage you to study it more on your own. Normally, I choose a purpose for each tea blend I formulate, selecting one or two primary herbs based on their affinities and effect on the body (e.g., chamomile and passionflower for sleep). I then choose one to three secondary herbs that can help activate the blend or make it taste better.

Before you formulate any teas on your own, please make a small cup of tea with each herb you want to work with and taste it first. This way, you'll be familiar with the flavor and strength of the herb before mixing a large batch together. Doing so will let you know how you need to balance the flavor and strength of the tea (often by adding a pleasant-tasting herb if your tea initially tastes overly bitter or earthy).

Note: When blending your own tea, the simplest method is to use "parts." YOU decide what that means in terms of your measurement size. If you want a small batch, you can use 1 teaspoon as 1 part. A larger batch could be ¼ cup as 1 part. You get the idea.

I encourage you to experiment with whatever herbs you have readily available and slowly expand your formulations as your knowledge and familiarity grow. What follows are a couple tea recipes to get you started, specifically geared toward easing symptoms you may experience when sick.

"I'm Sick" Tea Blend

1 part dried bee balm

1 part dried echinacea flower

2 parts dried ginger leaves (or fresh ginger root chunks)

2 parts dried mullein leaf

2 parts dried stinging nettle

(Optional: either 1-part dried licorice root or 2 parts dried marshmallow leaf)

Instructions:

Blend all herbs together and store in a glass jar until needed. Use 1 Tbsp of the blend per mug of hot water. Steep for at least 20 minutes and drink 2-3 cups a day.

Tummy Ache Tea Blend

1 part dried birch bark

2 parts dried or fresh ginger root

1-2 parts lemon (either dried peel or fresh chunks) OR 1-part dried peppermint

1-part dried thyme

Instructions:

Blend all herbs together and store in a glass jar until needed. Steep 1 Tbsp of tea in a mug of hot water and drink it slowly. This can help relieve pain from a stomach flu as well as a stomachache.

Note: Do NOT give this tea to a dog, as birch contains natural xylitol, which is toxic to dogs and can result in death.

Herbal Steams

Herbal steams are simple preparations that can make a big impact on your body. To make an herbal steam, choose herbs that have a strong scent that you can smell. This indicates their high volatile oil content. The volatile oils of certain plants can travel through steam (from a cup of tea or an herbal steam) into your sinuses to help break up thick mucus and allow you to breathe better. Bee balm, birch bark, cedar, lavender, lemon balm, oregano, peppermint, sage, sassafras, and thyme are all great herbs to try out. You can work with fresh herbs if you have them, but this will also work with dried herbs. This is an amazing remedy for a stopped-up nose!

Measure out 1-2 tablespoons of your herbal blend into a glass or ceramic bowl. Make sure you remove your glasses if you're wearing any and have a paper towel handy for when you're finished. Pour about a cup of boiling water over the herbs. Take a large dish towel and open it up, setting it atop the back of your head, and lean over the bowl. Breathe the steam in through your nose as best you can. After a few minutes you should start to notice things feeling more loose inside your nasal cavity. When the steam is slowing down or you feel ready, lift your head back up and blow your nose into the paper towel.

Don't forget to say, "Eeeew!" when you see how much has come out of your sinuses!

To learn more about performing an herbal steam, you can watch my short video on just that (referenced at the end of the book). Additionally, hanging a branch of cedar or eucalyptus when you take a hot, steamy shower can often perform the same function as the bowl steam.

If you need help flushing out your sinuses but cannot do an herbal steam, I suggest you get a Neti pot. You must use distilled or boiled (but not hot!) water with your Neti pot, rather than water from the tap (unless you have a filtration system installed).

Earaches and Ear Infections

While more common in children than in adults, adults can suffer from earaches and ear infections too, especially during allergy season or if they are prone to swimmer's ear. If you know someone dealing with an unexplained earache, I have a simple remedy that works great!

Mullein flower (*Verbascum thapsus*) is specific for earaches and ear infections. If you can pick enough of the flowers, you can make an infused oil with them (in combination with garlic). This remedy does not keep long-term, so I suggest if you make it yourself, you either only keep it for two weeks or store it in the fridge. Alternatively, you can also buy a premade version if you are unable to make it yourself.

Have your child or the person suffering from the earache lie on the couch on their side with the painful ear up. Warm the oil bottle in a small pan of hot water for a few minutes. (It is best warmed but will still work even if you don't warm it.) Put 4-5 drops in the affected person's ear. Have them lie there for at least 2 minutes while the oil makes its way into the ear canal. Then put a piece of cotton ball into their ear before they sit up so that when the oil drains out, it goes into the cotton ball rather than all over their shirt. Do this 2-3 times a day until the pain is gone.

Over time, often with trial and error, you will find methods and herbs that work for you and your family when you are sick or generally unwell. Hopefully, you'll heed my advice and stop drinking Schweppes Ginger Ale when you're home sick and instead get a bottle of ginger beer (made with real ginger chunks) or a bottle of kombucha to settle your stomach. And instead of having a can of Campbell's Soup, you'll grab some of your own homemade bone broth from the freezer and heat it up.

While it's important to take care of your body all the time, it certainly requires an increased amount of care and attention when you're sick or unwell. It's best to have some protocols in place for when you or a loved one does fall ill so you're not scrambling, trying to figure out what to do when sickness does strike. And if you're reading this while you're lying on your sofa, sick as a dog, know this: It's okay to rest and recharge. You'll feel better soon!

Chapter 24: Allergies

There are several different ways allergies can present themselves in our bodies. The most common one, and the one I'm now an expert at managing, is seasonal allergies (a.k.a., hay fever). Seasonal allergies typically flare up during springtime, when the birch, pine, and other wind-pollinated trees open up their cones and let their tree sperm fly out on the breeze, hoping to land on and fertilize female cones. Your body's immune system can only handle so much of an allergen before it becomes overloaded. The time it takes your body to react to an allergen you are sensitive to depends on your personal immune system, based on your general health, your stress levels, and your genetics.

As aptly stated on The School of Evolutionary Herbalism's website:

> Your body has a threshold for inflammation. You have a certain degree of tolerance—a buffer—substances you may be mildly intolerant to or even allergic to. This tends to apply more to intolerances than true allergies, but the concept is relevant to both. Essentially, your body has the capacity to handle a certain amount of inflammatory stimulus without expressing symptoms. Once that threshold is surpassed, symptoms appear. (Popham, 2025)

Other allergies, such as to bee stings or certain foods, can vary in their severity and change or develop as we age. Remember how I told you I'm allergic to cane sugar? That allergy only began after

I turned 40. You can bet your ass I was eating Twinkies and birthday cake aplenty when I was a kid. Now, not so much.

I'm also allergic to bees, an allergy I developed in adulthood as well. Thankfully, my reaction to a bee sting is mild; my heart rate drops, I feel nauseated, and I become woozy or faint for a few hours (when the sting goes untreated). Treatment for me is simple: I either take a Benadryl (which I recommend you keep on hand in case you or someone you live with has any kind of allergy) or I take a ton of stinging nettle tincture.

Before I tell you my allergy tincture recipe—the one that has saved me many times over from both mild bee stings and hay fever—I want to make sure you understand the difference between an intolerance and an allergy. Without going into great scientific detail, an **intolerance** typically refers to a food intolerance. When you're intolerant to a certain food or food group (such as dairy or wheat), the symptoms are mostly gastrointestinal. You may experience serious bloating, diarrhea, gas, stomach upset, sudden acne outbreaks, and even headaches after consuming a food you are intolerant to.

A food or substance **allergy** is far more serious and can land you in the hospital if you aren't careful to avoid it. An allergic reaction can be mild (such as my reaction to bee stings as described above), or it can be more serious, causing severe hives or anaphylaxis and requiring you to carry an EpiPen wherever you go. An EpiPen contains epinephrine, which counteracts histamines caused by a severe allergic reaction. It can save your life, but you need to know that the effects of the shot are only meant to keep you alive and support your body until you can get to a hospital for real treatment. It's meant to be a first-aid measure, not the only measure you depend on when experiencing anaphylactic shock.

It's important to note that some allergies may worsen over time. It's possible that someday my mild bee sting allergy could develop into full-blown anaphylactic shock, so I keep that in mind any time I accidentally make contact with a bee. Allergies can be deadly. I do not want you to test yours if they're serious, as doing so can be highly dangerous. Please seek advice from a medical professional if you're unsure what severity of allergy you have to a given allergen.

Allergy Tincture

2-3 parts stinging nettle tincture

2 parts goldenrod tincture

2 parts ground ivy tincture

2 parts mullein leaf tincture

1 part licorice root tincture

1 part pineapple core tincture

Instructions:

You can blend these herbs together in one big jar and tincture them with 100 proof (50%) ethanol, or you can tincture each separately and then blend them together. **NOTE**: If you suffer from serious high blood pressure problems, either use this remedy sparingly or omit the licorice root, as that plant can cause your blood pressure to go up in large enough doses.

During the time I am writing this book, I am still making my anti-allergy tincture to sell in my shop and at festivals, but I wanted to share my recipe with you because the day will inevitably come when I'm no longer making it to sell.

This recipe has served me incredibly well during allergy season for several years now. I truly rely on it when May rolls around, with it helping me avoid the dreaded "sneezy time." I add pineapple core because it's a source of bromelain, a constituent that works well against allergies when combined with the quercetin from the stinging nettle and goldenrod. It also helps the tincture taste better.

I can't sing the praises of stinging nettle enough for so many of its uses, with this tincture being the main one. Because my bee sting allergy is so mild, I can take about 3 droppers full of this tincture if I get stung and feel right as rain. I do this in conjunction with the application of a plantain poultice directly to the sting to ease itching, swelling, and pain. Always make sure you remove the stinger as soon as possible after being stung!

I cannot guarantee that this remedy will work for you. What I can tell you is that I have many customers who rely on this formula during hay fever season, as it helps relieve their many seasonal allergy symptoms, as it does mine. I hope it helps you too. And of course, remember that the best course of action is to simply avoid anything you are allergic to.

Chapter 25: Skin Issues

There are three main reasons why skin problems occur. Two of them are acute—normally temporary problems—and one is chronic.

The first acute skin issue you may experience is **contact dermatitis**. This occurs when your skin comes into contact with something you are allergic to, such as a new laundry detergent or poison ivy. This is always a temporary problem, so do not fret if you are experiencing this type of skin issue. As long as you identify the source of what you came into contact with and you cease further contact, the rash will eventually go away on its own with or without treatment.

The second type of acute skin issue is **fungal** in nature, resulting in infections such as ringworm and athlete's foot. As in the aforementioned category, this is also caused by a source that is external from your body. These types of infections can be contracted by touching an infected surface or animal that is carrying the fungus. Depending on how you go about treating it, this sort of infection can be quickly resolved or can linger for years. It generally requires treatment with some sort of fungicide to help your body remove the fungus completely. I would recommend black walnut leaf or hull tincture applied topically if you are treating this type of infection.

Skin issues caused by fungus are tricky, though. If you're regularly eating lots of sugary foods, you can end up with candida overload, which feeds the fungus on your skin from the sugar inside your body. It's paramount that you keep your skin dry as much as possible and reduce your sugar intake while you're treating any kind of fungal infection.

The third problem is chronic, the most difficult to fix, and takes the longest to develop: **skin problems which are related to your digestive tract**. Leaky gut or food allergies are the primary cause behind acne, eczema, psoriasis, and rosacea. Your digestive tract absorbs almost everything you consume, breaking "nutrients into small enough parts for your body to absorb and use for energy, growth, and cell repair" (National Institute of Diabetes and Digestive and Kidney Diseases, 2017).

If you eat a rock, it goes right through you because it isn't food. Alternatively, when you eat a carrot, your body breaks that down into its components, and the villi in your intestine absorb the vitamins (A, C, K, and everything else). It lets the fiber degrade and push its way out until everything useful has been extracted and there's nothing but a blob of waste (poop) that gets expelled.

Healing your gut lining and shifting to a whole foods diet, as outlined in the beginning of the book, will give your body the nutrients it needs to heal chronic skin issues, as the majority of skin conditions you may develop come about as a result of poor gut health and poor dietary choices. Think about it this way: Your eyes cannot see into your stomach; they can only see what is outside yourself. You look at your skin every day. So if something is wrong *inside* your body, how can your body let you know? By giving you symptoms where you can see them—on your skin!

I have included a link to a short quiz you can take that can give you some insight into the factors that contribute to leaky gut. If you are experiencing anxiety, autoimmune conditions, brain fog, diverticulitis/diverticulosis, eczema, GERD, IBS, or other skin issues, it is likely you have some degree of leaky gut. Again, if you want more in-depth guidance on healing your gut (and all the parts of your body your gut affects), please see my Gut Healing Protocol.

Your skin has three major layers. The outer layer serves as the protective barrier, which is why it's harder to cut into and takes more effort to rub moisture into. The second layer is the one that contains blood vessels and sweat glands. The third layer holds fat cells and cushions your organs (Yousef et al., 2024).

Your skin is thick enough that it repels water, and it's a good thing it does. It means your skin's not going to absorb all that scum from that pond you like to go swimming in during the summertime. *But* a percentage of everything that makes contact with your skin is absorbed into it.

Often, parabens, phthalates, and other chemical compounds are added to a wide range of cosmetics and skincare, mainly acting as preservatives. Although they continue to be widely used, these chemicals have been shown to disrupt the functioning of your body's endocrine system, which is the system that creates your body's hormones (Holland, 2024).

In addition to absorbing things that come into physical contact with your skin, your body absorbs anything you introduce into your digestive tract. The consumption of sugar leads to a spike in insulin levels, which in turn can increase the production of sebum, the oily substance that clogs pores and leads to acne (Pappas, 2009). This is why you tend to break out any time you eat pizza and ice cream with your friends.

Here's the cycle: You eat junk food or ultra-processed snacks and drinks (yes, that includes alcohol), which causes your skin to erupt in pimples. Then you go to the pharmacy and grab a zit cream that's full of toxic chemicals to try to treat the pimples you could have avoided simply by making better food choices. In turn, your skin may worsen from whatever topical you used. Stress from various factors in your life leads you to reach for your comfort food or drink, starting the cycle anew.

The more frequently this scenario plays out, the more toxic chemicals your body will be exposed to and absorb. Before you know it, you're 40 years old and facing a cancer diagnosis and an overactive histamine response, causing you to be allergic to just about everything you used to enjoy.

Contact Dermatitis

Contact dermatitis is not the same as eczema, though some dermatologists say it is for simplicity's sake. It is an eczema-like rash that occurs on part of your body as a result of touching something you are allergic to. This could result from using a certain laundry detergent (most of which are full of synthetic fragrances and chemicals that shouldn't be anywhere near the human body), from wearing a particular type of fabric, or from touching something briefly, such as poison ivy or a latex glove.

Anyone can experience contact dermatitis. The good news is that once you figure out what's causing the problem, it's easy to fix. I got contact dermatitis a couple of years ago after I let a friend use my washing machine. After their load was finished, I did a load of my own laundry a few hours later. Over the next few days I noticed small, square-ish, raised patches of skin on my neck and back, then a full-blown rash on my torso.

I went to my dermatologist in a panic. He claimed I had eczema and dispensed a steroid cream for me to apply to the itchy spots.

I rolled my eyes, but I took the cream to use for one night of relief on the rash before I was able to solve the problem myself.

It turned out I was allergic to the detergent my friend had used, and there was still some residue on the inside of the washing machine. I ran the washing machine with hot water and white vinegar twice to cleanse the machine before washing all my laundry again with the unscented, hypoallergenic laundry soap I make myself. My skin was on the mend by the next day, and the rash was completely gone within a week.

Athlete's Foot or Ringworm

A natural solution for a topical fungal infection is black walnut leaf or hull tincture applied topically as a liniment. Both black walnut leaves and the green hulls around the nuts are antifungal in nature. Make a tincture with the leaves or hulls (it will turn black). In 4 weeks, strain the solids out and use the tincture orally or topically. To apply to athlete's foot, soak a cotton ball with the tincture and apply to the affected area at least twice daily.

It's critical that you keep your feet dry as often as possible. Go barefoot the minute you are home from work and let your toes air out. You can put foot-drying powder inside your shoes. If you want to make your own herbal foot-drying powder, harvest some hemlock bark and dehydrate it. Grind the dehydrated bark into a powder and sprinkle some inside your shoes daily to help keep the insides dry and fresh.

Both of these conditions can also be helped by healing the candida overload inside your body. Those who don't suffer from an internal imbalance won't likely contract the foot fungus for very long. You're most likely to contract athlete's foot by touching the foot of another person who has it or by walking barefoot in wet public areas like showers or pools, as other people there may be carrying and spreading the fungus. Treating it and drying everything out is key.

Eczema

Eczema is a prime example of how gut dysbiosis affects the skin (Lee et al., 2018). I've been asked by hundreds of people how to heal their eczema, my own mother included. Mothers with infants ask me why their infant suddenly developed eczema after they switched from breast milk to baby formula. The same entreaties come from teenagers' parents when their child develops patches on their arms that do not seem to go away.

The sad truth is that the majority of people who say they want help healing their eczema will never do what it takes to solve the problem. How do you resolve and reverse your eczema? Stop eating the foods that are causing it, heal your gut lining, and stop using products that trigger contact dermatitis. You need to decide what is more important to you. Is the pleasure you derive from having certain foods and beverages—your love of sourdough bread or your addiction to Mountain Dew—worth the pain and embarrassment your eczema causes you?

Now, when an infant shows signs of eczema, I can completely understand a parent's concern. If you had to start feeding your baby formula for any number of reasons, there's no shame in that. However, if your baby is showing eczema on their skin, I would advise you to try a different brand or type of formula as soon as possible. Goat milk baby formula would be my first choice as an alternative to breast milk since it is the closest substitute. But you'll have to do what's best for you and your baby, finding the variety of formula they can eat without triggering the eczema rash.

If an infant is showing signs of eczema and is breastfed, it tells me that the mother is most likely eating something that is causing her baby's eczema. If you are a mother in such a position, take a look at your diet; know that everything you eat is going into your baby's body via your breast milk. Is there an inflammatory food that sticks out to you, or perhaps a processed food with a lot of chemical dyes or flavorings in it that you have been eating? You will need to experiment with eliminating one food or drink at a time for at least one week each to see how it affects your baby.

In any case, if your baby is showing signs of eczema, an infant probiotic can help regulate your baby's microbiome—both gut and skin. Look for a high-quality liquid probiotic supplement that you can give your baby every day, like Lovebug Baby Probiotic Drops. It can also help if you are taking a good supplement, like Silver Fern™ Ultimate Probiotic, especially while you're breastfeeding.

Psoriasis

Another common skin problem many people face is psoriasis, which is generally caused by a combination of leaky gut and stress (Ely, 2018). Some other common causes of psoriasis are alcohol consumption, smoking, sunburns or cuts, and sometimes medications, such as beta blockers (used to treat heart conditions), lithium (used to treat bipolar disorder), and prednisone (a steroid).

Reducing your stress levels is a key component of managing psoriasis. However, if the only way you can deal with your stress is through an addiction (food, alcohol, tobacco, or recreational drugs), you will not be solving the problem and can make your skin condition significantly worse. It's necessary that you utilize healthy options for stress relief rather than succumbing to a food or substance addiction if you want to see real improvement in your condition.

I recently discovered, almost completely by accident, that rubbing the inside of a banana peel on psoriasis-affected skin stops the itching for up to six hours and helps heal the skin tissue. Doing this every day and showering with a natural, healing shampoo at least three times a week has nearly cured the condition in one client of mine. If you're experiencing psoriasis, I recommend you use a psoriasis-specific shampoo and conditioner every 2-3 days, like the set made by Wild Naturals.

There are medications your doctor can give you to help treat your psoriasis, but in many cases, a steroid shot or cream is only going to temporarily relieve your symptoms. To learn more about natural solutions, you can watch my short video on how I helped my client heal their psoriasis (linked in the Additional Resources section at the end of the book).

Below is a recipe for an herbal salve you can make that helps ease itching caused by eczema, psoriasis, and issues such as insect bites or stings:

Itch Salve Recipe

¼ cup calendula-infused oil

¼ cup plantain-infused oil

¼ cup St. John's wort-infused oil

3 Tbsp beeswax pellets

20 drops chamomile essential oil

Instructions:

Combine your infused oils and beeswax in a bowl atop a pot that's filled halfway with water to use as a double boiler system. Cook on medium heat until steam has melted all the beeswax. Turn off the heat and add your chamomile essential oil. Pour the mixture into glass or metal containers. This will make a pretty big batch of salve and will last two years if kept in a cool, dark place. Apply as needed to itchy skin or rashes.

Rosacea

Rosacea is most often caused by leaky gut or SIBO (small intestinal bacterial overgrowth) (Wang & Chi, 2021). It's a prime example of how gut dysbiosis can directly affect your skin. I was diagnosed with rosacea in 2020, but I have since healed it completely by quitting alcohol and healing my gut microbiome.

When I got my diagnosis, I was told that the rosacea I had was mainly caused by an overgrowth of demodex mites. DO NOT GOOGLE pictures of demodex mites; they are a thing of nightmares. Suffice it to say, they are microscopic mites that live inside your hair follicles (mainly your eyebrows and eyelashes) that come out at night to mate and poop on your face.

A normal count of mites on the face is about 10-15 per person. When your gut is out of whack (dysbiosis), conditions on your skin are *perfect* to feed the mites all the sugary skin cells they could dream of. This causes rosacea. People with rosacea have upwards of 45-50 mites in their eyebrows and eyelashes, and sometimes the mites can travel across the face to other hair follicles on the skin.

Now that you know what's happening, I bet you can't WAIT to heal your gut!

Avoiding dairy is usually the first step to resolving rosacea. When I was healing my gut, I avoided my triggers, which were dairy products and alcohol. Any time I ate cow dairy, the blood vessels in my nose would start to turn red again, so I simply started avoiding eating it. Nowadays, I'm so used to going without cow dairy I don't even think of it except during ice cream season. In the summer I carry a Lactaid capsule with me just in case I get a hankering for ice cream. The Lactaid really does the trick, but I still don't indulge in ice cream very often because 1) I don't want to push my luck and 2) the sugar content of ice cream will do my gut and skin microbiomes just as much harm as the dairy.

General Skincare

Eating the right foods to maintain healthy skin is critical. This includes lots of fruits and vegetables, especially those high in vitamin C, since it helps hold your skin together. Without sufficient levels of vitamin C, your scar tissue can degrade, and your skin won't be able to properly heal itself.

Another important nutrient for skin health is DHA, which is found in omega-3 fatty acids. You mainly derive DHA from eating fish. Most people have an abundance of omega-6 fatty acids in their diet but are not balancing them out with enough omega-3. This imbalance is one of the contributing factors in developing skin problems, such as dry skin, frequent sunburns, and even acne. My suggestion is to eat a can of sardines (or other fatty fish, such as cod, mackerel, salmon, sardines, trout, or tuna) at least twice a week. Alternatively, you can take a high-quality supplement of either fish oil or algae oil.

Cleanse your skin daily with a gentle cream cleanser and exfoliate once a week with a gentle, organic exfoliating scrub. Every morning, I wash my face with witch hazel extract that I make myself. Use a moisturizer on your face at night and sunscreen on your face during the day. Always wear a good-quality, reef-safe sunscreen on your face daily. You also want to have one that's safe to use on your body as well. The main ingredient you are looking for is zinc oxide; the fewer the ingredients in your sunscreen, the better.

I use a gua sha tool every morning on my face and neck (after jumping up and down and moving my arms around for a few seconds) in order to help drain lymphatic fluid naturally. In order for the tool to glide smoothly, I blend my own face oil with argan oil as a base plus carrot seed oil, frankincense oil, rosehip seed oil, and sea buckthorn seed oil. You can get my handmade Aging Face Oil Blend on my online shop.

I make myself a smoothie every day (usually before lunchtime) with a small handful of black grapes, blueberries, cherries, cranberries, strawberries, and spinach (all frozen). I then add some almond or coconut milk, 100% juice (such as acai, cherry, or pomegranate), a small shake of ground clove powder, and a teaspoon of bee pollen.

Additionally, I add acai powder, cacao powder, hemp seed protein powder (hemp is the only plant that has complete protein like whey, so it is a good substitute if you are intolerant to whey), kelp powder, maca powder, moringa powder, flax seeds, two Brazil nuts, and some ginger (fresh if I have it, powdered if not).

Both oral and topical collagen can help prevent skin aging (Al-Atif, 2022). I found a powdered collagen that includes all four types of collagen as well as hyaluronic acid, so I don't need to buy a different supplement for each one. I add 1-2 tbsp of collagen powder to my daily smoothie, but you can take it in applesauce or something else if you prefer.

A warning from me to you: I tried colostrum supplements because I thought they'd help my skin and hair, but they ended up making me nauseated all day, every day. I switched back to regular collagen and haven't had a problem since.

Reducing the Appearance of Scars

The two herbs I utilize most often to help with healing scar tissue are calendula-infused oil (Jahdi et al., 2018) and St. John's wort-infused oil (Samadi et al., 2010). I prefer using a high-quality olive oil for most of my infusions, but if you want to make something specifically for delicate skin or your face, I recommend argan or almond oil (both of which contain skin-healing vitamin E). Gotu kola (*Centella asiatica*) can also be made into an infused oil to reduce scar tissue when applied topically.

Sunburns and Heat Rashes

Always go for a cooling remedy in the case of burns or rashes. Aloe vera is my number one go-to. It's easy to keep an aloe plant alive for years on a windowsill with minimal watering. You can also buy aloe gel at most stores in the summertime, storing it in your bathroom closet for several years to use as needed.

Another great remedy for sunburns is cleavers juice. Cleavers (*Gallium aparine*) is a plant I forage in the early spring. I pick bunches and bunches of it and put it into a blender with some water. Then I blend it and pour the mush through cheesecloth into a jar. Pour this green juice into ice cube trays for easy access. They will keep for up to a year in your freezer. If you get sunburned, simply grab a cleavers cube and apply it to the affected skin. It will cool and heal the burn simultaneously.

Always wear sunscreen! Badger Mineral Sunscreen is a good option if you have not found one yet. Again, zinc oxide is the main ingredient you want to look for in an environmentally safe and non-toxic sunscreen. If possible, find a local herbalist who makes their own so you can buy high-quality skincare and support a small business at the same time.

St. John's Wort oil applied topically can help heal the damaged sunburned skin once the bubbling or swelling has gone down. Use caution with this herb, however, as if you have it on your skin topically BEFORE you go outside (or if you are taking it internally for some reason) it can actually cause your skin to get sunburned even worse than normal.

Cherry Angiomas

If you are a white person over the age of 30, you probably have a few cherry angiomas on your skin. They look like little, mini raised moles, but they are bright red rather than a shade of brown. They're a normal part of European heritage and are harmless. But when you go from having a few dozen across your body to hundreds, it sounds an alarm!

I'm not sure whether there is any scientific proof of the connection between kelp/seaweed consumption and cherry angiomas, but I noticed the correlation in my own body. There's a fairly good chance you may notice it in yours too if you begin taking kelp. When I stopped taking kelp powder for a time, I noticed that the angiomas went from appearing at a normal rate to wildly proliferating. To help keep the cherry angiomas at bay, I add ¼ tsp kelp powder to my daily smoothie.

How to Remove a Wart or Mole

It is SO easy to remove a wart! I use the same process for removing a mole, though it works best on the kind of mole that has a distinctly raised edge rather than a slightly raised freckle.

Supplies you will need: cotton balls, raw apple cider vinegar, and either Band-Aids or medical tape.

Method: Take a cotton ball and pull a small piece off, large enough to cover the mole or wart. Soak it in raw apple cider vinegar and squeeze out a little of the excess so it isn't dripping. Set it carefully atop the mole or wart and cover it with a band-aid or medical tape so it is attached to the surrounding skin. Change this out at least twice a day. It works great if you can do it at night before bed but will work even faster if you can keep the bandage on day and night. Within a week the mole or wart should turn black, dry up, and fall off.

Warning: This method may sting or burn a bit while the apple cider vinegar is in contact with your skin. The last time I used this method, the acidic ACV burned the skin around the mole I was removing, so it was angry and red for several days, even after the mole fell off. Rubbing some aloe vera gel on the skin helped soothe it. Don't do this for more than two weeks. If it hasn't worked within two weeks, you need to seek a different method (and possibly help from a doctor).

Your skin is one of your most vital organs, as it protects you from a myriad of external contaminants you encounter in day-to-day life. Although it keeps many bad things out, its health is greatly affected by what you put into your body. Skin issues without a clear cause, and especially the chronic kind, can often be traced back to gut dysbiosis. If you're having recurrent skin issues, it may be time to evaluate what is going on internally.

While it serves as an effective barrier, your skin does absorb a percentage of (almost) everything you come into physical contact with. Products that contain known irritants and toxins should be avoided whenever possible to avoid allergic reactions, contact dermatitis, endocrine (hormone) disruption, and a host of other issues.

Now that we've discussed your skin—its composition, the gut-skin connection, common issues, natural solutions, and general skincare—it's time we delve even further into a topic we began to touch on in this chapter: your hormones and the effects of endocrine disruptors. To fully take control of your health, you need to understand the role of your hormones, how to regulate them, and the disruptors to avoid.

Chapter 26: Hormone Imbalances

Your hormones dictate a great number of functions in your body: how tall you get, how much you weigh, how large your sexual organs are and how they function, how your blood sugar is regulated, your body temperature, and much more (Johns Hopkins Medicine, 2019). Whether your hormones are balanced is determined largely by your diet, exercise levels, and age. Once you've changed your relationship with food and are treating your body like the sacred temple it truly is, you will be less likely to suffer imbalances that are food-related.

Your body depends on receiving a delicate balance of nutrients in order to create the right amounts of each hormone. Your diet has a LOT to do with whether your hormones are balanced or are out of whack. You also need to remember to drink enough water daily, especially if you're a woman who's on her period; losing blood means you're losing iron and water.

One of the most common causes of PMS is a deficiency in vitamin B2, magnesium, and zinc (Abdi et al., 2019). You're not deficient in Vitex or red clover—you're deficient in NUTRIENTS. I bring up this point to demonstrate how nutrient intake directly affects hormonal balance. Herbs can aid you in balancing your hormones, but they cannot make up for a nutritional deficiency; nothing can other than getting the missing nutrient through your diet or through supplementation.

In some ways, your body functions as a machine. It gets you from point A to point B, but only when you give it the fuel it needs to function and run properly. Many people take better care of their cars than they do their own bodies. Don't be like them. If you neglect your body for too long, not performing regular maintenance, it will eventually break down, landing you in the metaphorical repair shop—the hospital.

I want to remind you here that I'm an herbalist, not an endocrinologist or a doctor. I'll refer you to some helpful resources at the end of this section that I recommend you print out and put on your bookshelf. They are on mine, and I refer back to them frequently, referencing authors who have expertise in their specific fields.

In the following chapters, we'll cover herbal hormone support for both women and men, including some fantastic resources where you can do further, in-depth reading. But, more important than herbal support, let's start with prevention.

In the previous chapter, we began our discussion on endocrine disruptors; now, let's expand on the topic. **Endocrine disruptors** are chemicals found in thousands of household products and even some clothing, which are absorbed through the skin or breathed in when you are near them. They are also found in a disturbingly high number of skincare products as well as plastics (National Institute of Environmental Health Sciences, 2024). I know you love your Tupperware, but it's part of the problem.

Endocrine disruptors DISRUPT YOUR ENDOCRINE SYSTEM, which is the thing inside your body that regulates your hormones. Steering clear of these chemicals is step one to preventing damage to your endocrine system as well as your other organ systems. How can you avoid them when they're in almost every body care and household cleaning product you find at the store? In all honesty, it's ridiculously easy to make your own effective cleaning products.

If you occasionally need to use something stronger, you can. I get it; I've been there too. But if the majority of the cleaning you do at home is done with cleaning agents that do not expose your endocrine system to various toxins, you're avoiding *serious* health risks. Such risks include developmental problems, immune system problems, metabolic issues, neurological problems, reproductive issues, and cancer (U.S. Environmental Protection Agency, 2024).

Here are a few easy recipes (that I've been using for years) to get you started:

Homemade Laundry Soap

1 bar of unscented goat milk soap, grated

1 cup Borax powder

1 cup washing soda

Instructions:

Use a bell grater to grate the soap into a big bowl. Add the other dry ingredients and whisk together until combined. That's it! I keep mine in an old trail mix jar with a teaspoon to scoop it out. Use 1-2 teaspoons of this per load, washing the load on warm so that the soap chunks dissolve.

When grating the soap, you'll end up with a small chunk at the end that you can't really grate; otherwise, you'll rip your knuckles apart on the grater. I suggest you save this and either use it to make more hand soap or save up a bunch and put them into a crocheted soap saver pouch to use in the shower.

Instead of dryer sheets, you can either use wool dryer balls or wad up a piece of aluminum foil into a ball and toss it into the dryer with your clothes. The foil will attract the static so you don't get shocked when you go to fold your clothes. The more you start wearing clothing made with natural fibers, the less static you'll experience out of the dryer.

Wool and linen clothes should be air-dried on a rack. Your remaining clothes should be dried on a line outdoors for as much of the year as possible. Doing so will help your clothes last longer (and save on your electricity bill).

Homemade Hand Soap

½ a bar of natural soap

2 quarts of water

Instructions:

Get yourself a large jug—a gallon-size container if you can. This is where you will store your hand soap. Glass is always best, but plastic will do.

Grate half a bar of soap (a natural one you can buy from someone at your local farmer's market is ideal) with a bell grater into a bowl. Combine it with two quarts of water in a saucepan. Cook on low for about 45 minutes to 1 hour, stirring occasionally, until all the soap has fully dissolved.

Cool the mixture before pouring it into your container. Use this to refill all the hand soap dispensers in your house. If you want to use a foaming dispenser, put a little of this soap into the bottle and fill the rest with water.

Yep, that's it! The hand soap you buy from the store may suds up a little better than this does, but this recipe is free of toxic ingredients and works just fine to clean your hands. What a racket the soap industry is, eh?

I know I keep hammering this point home, but I'm going to say it again: Your hormones are absolutely affected by your diet. Eating too much sodium can increase your cortisol levels, eating too many saturated fats can interrupt your leptin signals (increasing your chances of obesity), and eating too much sugar can negatively impact your insulin levels (The Institute for Functional Medicine, 2025).

If you're losing hair, having irregular menstruation, or experiencing twitchy legs at night, you are likely suffering from a hormone imbalance. In any of these instances, I would recommend you eat beef, calf, or lamb liver with onions once a week. A portion that's about the size of your palm is enough. This is one of the easiest ways to get the minerals your body needs—straight from a whole food source. If your body truly needs the vitamins and minerals found in liver, you probably won't mind the taste.

On days you don't eat liver, you can take a teaspoon of cod liver oil. I also take a trace mineral supplement on most of the days I don't eat liver to help support iron absorption and distribution. In a pinch, I will take a capsule of Hema-Plex, but supplementing more iron isn't usually necessary. If you are unable to eat liver, I would recommend you try Pure Encapsulations Mineral Complex, which has worked well for me and also includes copper!

You're probably not anemic because of low iron. In fact, most people get more than enough iron from their diet. The real issue is getting iron to move to the right places in your body; that's where trace minerals come in. The top six vital minerals that affect hormone balance in women are calcium, iodine, iron, magnesium, selenium, and zinc (Kapper et al., 2024). Your body needs sufficient quantities of ALL of these trace minerals in order for it (and your hormones) to function properly. Hormone imbalances can manifest as PMS, mood swings, cravings, insomnia, and more (West Bengal Chemical Industries Limited, 2025).

So why do I keep talking about liver? Because it's one of the most powerful sources of trace minerals in the entire food web. Your body needs cobalt, copper, manganese, iron, selenium, and zinc—all of which are found in liver—to maintain internal balance and keep your whole system running smoothly. If I have a poor night's sleep, I make sure to eat some beef liver with my dinner the next day, after which I am welcomed with a good night's sleep.

Being on **hormonal birth control** for more than six months consecutively—whether it's the pill, the shot, the patch, the hormonal IUD, or whatever is dripping synthetic hormones into your system—can affect your body (and brain) for years even after you stop taking it. While there haven't been any long-term scientific studies done on the effects of birth control on women (for longer than 10 years at a time), there is a lot of anecdotal evidence that suggests it takes anywhere from a few months to several years for a woman's body to fully readjust and rebalance her hormones once she ceases taking hormonal birth control.

Like many women, I was on hormonal birth control for a *long* time—17 years to be exact. Does that number sound familiar? It correlates precisely with the amount of time I was suffering from chronic candida. Yes, birth control affects the health of the inside of your vagina as much as it affects your mood and ability to conceive.

Many doctors will prescribe birth control as a means to balance your hormones if you're experiencing PCOS, irregular periods, or a number of other menstrual-related symptoms, no matter what your age is. This is mainly because modern Western doctors are not trained to resolve the root cause of the problem, which in many cases is related to the woman's diet and a lack of certain minerals. Instead, it's easier to simply prescribe birth control as an all-purpose panacea for any "women's problem" and allow the woman to sort out her side effects later.

While I completely understand the desire to have sex with your partner without becoming pregnant, hormonal birth control is not the only answer. There are ways to track your fertility and other methods of contraception that won't negatively impact your body, mental health, and personality. The Fertility Awareness Method, if adhered to correctly, is an amazing tool for women to understand their bodies and take control of their reproduction.

Any time you want to have sex during your body's fertile window, the span of 4-5 days when your body can conceive, you can use another form of birth control such as condoms or spermicide. All the while, you're tracking your body's temperature daily and staying aware of what phase of your cycle you're in. This system is outlined perfectly in the book *Taking Charge of Your Fertility*, a must-read for any woman under the age of 45.

Returning back to the harms of hormonal birth control, there have been studies written on a subject I am all too familiar with: how birth control can affect who you choose as your life partner (Alvergne & Lummaa, 2010; Cobey et al., 2015; Hill, 2020;

Taylor, 2020). In her book, *This is Your Brain on Birth Control*, Sarah E. Hill, an avid researcher and writer on hormones and birth control, states

> Although many of us think of hormones as something that "happen" to us, that isn't quite right. You are your hormones. They help to form your very identity, the beliefs you have about yourself, and your behaviors. So going on and off the pill can change your very sense of who you are. It can prompt a change in identity—one that's seemingly common but those scientists haven't fully explored yet. (2019)

I was on the pill when I met the man who would become my first husband. I remember the first time I ever saw him at a party we were both attending. My first thought when I laid eyes on him was, "I can do better."

Unfortunately, I'm serious. That was probably my intuition asking me, "What the hell are you thinking?!" But I didn't listen. I remember being attracted to him even though I wasn't quite sure why, and as such overlooking our total incompatibility. Hormonal birth control altered my hormones, thus altering my hormonal response and attraction to certain people. It changed the way my body responded to pheromones. It didn't help that I was also mentally struggling back then, but I know that the Pill was responsible for my sexual attraction to someone who was so wrong for me.

It is my belief that the relationship wouldn't have happened without the emotional and mental changes I experienced from being on birth control. I know it has its place; don't get me wrong. Birth control gave me the luxury of sexual freedom. But I would have sought alternative options if I had known back then how much it would affect the rest of my life.

Please remember (and remind your daughters) how important it is to spend time with your intended spouse while OFF hormonal birth control before taking the plunge into marriage. Otherwise, you won't be able to ascertain whether your feelings and attraction are due to the influence birth control has on your hormones. If you're not diligent, you could be in for a rude awakening down the road. Learn from my experience and save yourself time and pain.

Hormone imbalances can arise from multiple different factors, including diet, endocrine disruption, and hormonal birth control. Exposure to endocrine-disrupting chemicals is a significant and growing risk to the average person, especially those people living in countries without strict rules and regulations governing the use of such chemicals. Although it may seem a daunting task to avoid hormone-disrupting ingredients, we have gone over some very simple and affordable ways to do so in this chapter.

Now that you're more aware of what to look out for and avoid as well as the important part diet plays in hormonal balance, we will cover hormonal support for both women and men, respectively. Additionally, we will discuss the hormones that most greatly impact each sex, common hormonal issues faced by each, and natural solutions that can gently correct imbalances.

Chapter 27: Herbal Support for Women

Before we get into herbal remedies and support, we need to cover the primary hormones that affect a woman's health. Women have two major hormones that have the most impact on their fertility, mood, and menstrual cycle: **estrogen** and **progesterone** (and, to a lesser extent, testosterone). This is the case for the average woman's body. If you have had a hysterectomy, a thyroidectomy, or any other major surgery affecting your female parts, your body may behave a little differently in terms of hormone production and regulation.

If you're still young enough that you get your period regularly, the easiest way to remember estrogen and progesterone is that during the first half of your cycle (before your peak fertility window), your body produces more **estrogen** and rides the high of feeling freaking fantastic. You love the way you look, you have more energy, and you might even be a little horny.

Then your egg drops, and you experience your **fertile window**: the 4-6 days in the middle of your cycle when your body is able to get pregnant. Yes, contrary to what school probably taught you, you can only get pregnant during this time frame of your cycle. This is why tracking your fertility (or the Fertility Awareness Method) is used by many women. The challenging thing is that during your fertile window, your body is horny as hell. Biologically, it's saying, "I want to make babies!" So you have to remember that these two things, your time of peak fertility and when you feel most aroused, typically correspond.

After your fertile window ends, your **progesterone** levels rise. You start to feel PMS coming on, you may gain a little weight or feel bloated, you want to eat comfort foods or chocolate, and you may dislike the way you look in the mirror. This is the moody phase of your cycle. It sucks, but it is natural. Typically, progesterone is at its peak the day before your period arrives. This is when you tell your boyfriend to leave you alone because leaving his beard hair all over the mirror after he shaves has pissed you off for the *last time.*

Another hormone I'm sure you've heard of is **testosterone**. It is much higher in men than in women, but it is present in women too. Women with high testosterone levels can end up growing hair in unusual places (such as their chest or chin) and may have a higher sex drive than a woman with lower testosterone levels. They may also experience acne or oily skin, thin hair atop their heads, irregular periods, or potentially even develop PCOS (polycystic ovarian syndrome).

PMS (premenstrual syndrome) is a sign of too much estrogen in the body, which can cause irritability, cravings, mood swings, breast tenderness, etc. It can be helped immensely by supplementing vitamin B6, B12, magnesium, and zinc, along with eating a healthy, wheat-free diet. Herbs that can help manage PMS symptoms and cramps include lady's mantle, lemon balm, red clover, and Vitex.

PMDD (premenstrual dysphoric disorder) is a much more serious and rarer disorder that is a sign of too much progesterone in the body. It can cause heightened anxiety, deep depression, increased irritability, sudden teary outbursts, and suicidal thoughts. You do NOT want to take Vitex if you're dealing with this disorder, as it will exacerbate the issue. Red clover may be an option for support, but again, getting the right balance of minerals is essential to effectively regulating your hormones. B vitamins can potentially support PMDD, with foods such as beans, peas, and most meats being abundant in B vitamins. Zinc can be a good option as well and can be found in many foods, including beef, eggs, oysters, poultry, and pumpkin seeds.

Supplementing with magnesium is critical for women, particularly as we get older and enter perimenopause and menopause. The amount of magnesium present in our blood decreases as we age and can cause thyroid imbalances (Kolanu et al., 2020). Magnesium is essential for hundreds of processes inside the human body. It contributes to a healthy nervous system, proper muscle function, and strong bones and teeth. Additionally, it helps break down your food into nutrients, which is vital for maintaining good gut health.

Magnesium bisglycinate is the best supplement you can take to increase your magnesium. You will want to take a 100 mg capsule every day, 4-5 times over the course of the day (not all at once). This particular supplement is beneficial for almost *everyone*, not just those suffering from menstrual disorders. In terms of women's health and hormones, having sufficient magnesium in the body will contribute to better sleep, lowered stress, fewer mood swings, reduced cramping and bloating, and fewer menstrual-related headaches (Harcourt, 2024).

What follows is a list of herbs you should be aware of when trying to balance your hormones. This is simply a place to start your research, not an exhaustive list. *Not to be taken if you are pregnant or nursing! *

Hormone-balancing herbs:

Chasteberry *(Vitex agnus-castus)*: If you're a woman googling natural hormone-balancing herbs, one of the first things to come up is going to be chasteberry (also commonly known as Vitex). Without going into a deep herbal lesson, this is what you should remember: Vitex increases progesterone, not estrogen. The most common cause of PMS symptoms (and some other common problems in women) is a deficiency of progesterone in the body. If this is the case for you, Vitex may help decrease your PMS symptoms by increasing progesterone. If, however, you have an abundance of progesterone, taking Vitex could have an adverse effect on your cycle and hormones. (If you aren't sure which of your hormones are out of balance, don't just guess! Get a blood test from your doctor to help you decide which foods and herbs can help balance your hormones.)

Vitex is a Mediterranean plant, but I have one growing in my backyard here in Connecticut. It is happier during summers when we have a drought and everything else is dying of heat exhaustion, but it does do okay with some rain. Vitex is hardy in Zones 6-9, so it does better in the Southern United States than in the North.

Evening primrose *(Oenothera biennis)*: Here, I'm talking about the evening primrose oil supplements you can buy from the store or online. Evening primrose contains GLA, which can help reduce PMS, breast pain, and skin conditions such as eczema. Evening primrose oil can also help slightly increase the natural lubrication inside the vagina. If you're dealing with vaginal dryness, you can buy some evening primrose oil (or pop some capsules with a pin) and rub a little oil inside the vaginal canal. This needs to be done every day, and you shouldn't expect results for at least two weeks.

Evening primrose oil must be extracted from the plant's seeds via mechanical means, so it isn't something most people can make at home. There are millions of tiny black seeds on a dried evening primrose plant. You can get the omega-6 GLA (gamma linoleic acid) content from directly eating the seeds if you don't wish to take a supplement. However, I find it easier to take a capsule rather than spend weeks trying to forage enough of the seeds to get the quantity I need.

Even though GLA is an omega-6 fatty acid, it's not the same as the omega-6s most people get from consuming vegetable oils. If you're also taking a DHA or fish oil supplement, you should take it a few hours before or after your evening primrose supplement because they are both absorbed through the same pathways inside your body. If taken at the same time, they will compete for which one gets absorbed. To learn more about evening primrose, you can watch my short video lesson (linked in the Additional Resources section at the end of the book).

Hops *(Humulus lupulus)*: Hops contains phytoestrogens and helps raise estrogen levels in both men and women (which is why I usually tell men that if they want to keep their high sex drive, they had better stay away from IPAs). It also acts as a powerful nervine and sleep aid (which is why you get sleepy after drinking beer). It's very bitter (which makes it cooling) and works best for people with a hot, damp constitution who struggle with poor digestion and insomnia. I suggest taking it as a tincture because the tea tastes very bitter, although the tea can also help aid digestion.

Red clover *(Trifolium pratense)*: Red clover is one of my favorite wild foods to eat, and for good reason—it's full of calcium, chromium, magnesium, niacin, phosphorus, potassium, thiamine, and vitamin C. Red clover contains phytoestrogens, which are plant compounds that mimic estrogen in the human body (Beck et al., 2005).

If your estrogen receptors are not creating enough estrogen, red clover can supplement the missing estrogen parts with its phytoestrogens. If your receptors are producing too much estrogen, red clover can take the place of some of the human estrogen and replace it with its own phytoestrogens, which are not as strong as human estrogen. Either way, red clover helps balance the existing estrogen in your body.

When foraging red clover, I eat the flowers with the few leaves near the top. However, you don't get the estrogen-balancing effects by simply eating this plant (unless you eat around a pound a day, which no one wants to do). For it to be most effective, you need to make the flowers into a tea or tincture. Every woman's needs are different, so if you choose to try red clover for its hormone-balancing properties, I suggest you start with a low dose to see how it affects you. I tested it for the first time two years ago, taking a half dropperful of tincture every day for about a week. By day 6, I got my period two weeks earlier than expected.

Continually picking red clover from the same patch encourages the plant to produce more. This means I will often be harvesting red clover flowers from early July through November for as long as temperatures stay above freezing (in Northern Zones, such as Zones 3-6). To learn more about red clover, you can watch my short video lesson (linked in the Additional Resources section at the end of the book).

Other herbs that you will want to research for hormone support are black cohosh, cramp bark, lady's mantle, and red raspberry leaf. Black cohosh root can help with cramping, spasms, and hot flashes. I have successfully taken black cohosh root tincture (that I made myself) for menstrual cramps, and it works like a charm! I think it's pretty obvious what cramp bark helps with: cramping. Lady's mantle serves as a gentle hormone-balancing herb (which can be grown easily in your garden). Red raspberry leaf can help with cramping and toning the uterus.

Despite claims to the contrary, I have found no evidence of either dong quai (Hirata et al., 1997) or wild yam (EBSCO CAM Review Board, 2024; Komesaroff et al., 2001) having any actual effect on the uterus or hormones, other than possibly helping with cramping. As far as I have read, these two herbs were touted as cure-alls for women's hormonal health as progesterone-balancing herbs way back in the 1980s due to a misunderstanding of the science of extracting estrogen from plants. The myth became popular and has been perpetuated ever since with no scientific evidence or truth. Therefore, I do not recommend "wild yam cream," no matter how viral and popular it is on the internet.

Happy Uterus Tea (for women who still menstruate)

2 parts lady's mantle

2 parts lemon balm

2 parts red raspberry leaf

1 part marshmallow leaf

1 part red clover blossom

Instructions:

Combine ingredients in a blender and pulse for a few seconds. Use 1 Tbsp of tea blend per 8 oz of hot water. Cover the cup with a lid or a small saucer while it steeps for ~15 minutes. Improve the taste by adding your desired amount of honey.

Menopause

Most women start menstruating around age 12-13 and stop menstruating around age 50-55. Perimenopause can begin as early as age 35 in women. It's the stage of life between a woman's reproductive years and the cessation of egg production. Menopause is the period of your life after you have stopped menstruating—basically the "Crone" part of your Maiden-Mother-Crone cycle.

This archetype is based on the ancient spiritual belief that women have three major phases during their life: the Maiden, when she is pure and free—untouched by man; the Mother, when she is pregnant or in her child-bearing years; and the Crone, the time past child-bearing age when her lived experience makes her a source of wisdom in her community and to younger women. During your Crone phase, you step into your power as a confident older woman who has been through the rigors of life and is now fully in control of her own destiny.

The next few pages were written by my friend Layne Whitley, who is a women's menopause and alcohol-free life coach and herbalist. Because I am not personally in perimenopause yet, and I know a lot of my readers are either in it or already on the other side of it, I asked her if she would write an entry on menopause in this chapter. I know you'll find her insights helpful, and I encourage you to seek out her coaching services if you're in need of support during your menopause journey.

Turning My Menopause Tornado into Service for Others

My first menopause coaching client was myself. I have been a certified life coach since 2007, specializing in alcohol-free lifestyle coaching. Today, I coach women through the challenging life chapter that is menopause, without them using the crutch of alcohol. But before I reached this point in my journey, I had to learn how to coach myself through menopause because I was falling apart!

I realized that I was out there on my own with my peri-, mid-, and post-menopause journey. My awakening to this challenging revelation began when a doctor told me—in the first 5 minutes of meeting each other—that I should have my uterus removed because of some cysts. They were causing my body to excessively bleed, resulting in anemia, fatigue, and other problems. On my own, I discovered that cysts were often part of perimenopause.

I was both irritated and worried by this suggestion from a new doctor who did not even know my name yet. I asked the doctor, "Aside from a hysterectomy, aren't there any other options to help this issue that I could try first? Like changing my diet or taking supplements before conducting a major, life-changing surgery?"

His quiet, sheepish response somewhat surprised me: "Yes."

That was the green light I needed. I dove into learning more about the foods that could help my uterus. Guess what? A simple diet shift helped my issue. This fueled my desire to learn more in order to better coach myself through these life changes.

I had to learn how to do this because I was also discovering that perimenopause was making me INSANE. No one warned me; no one prepared me. I found myself clenching and shaking my fist at other drivers when someone cut me off on the highway. I had to hold back from expletives if the checkout person was taking too long. Suddenly, I had a temper and inappropriate knee-jerk reactions that I was fighting hard to suppress.

I could feel the cortisol coursing through my body, but I didn't know what it was at the time. I just felt incredibly stressed out, with very low coping skills. Lack of coping skills also manifested in severe mood swings. I dearly love animals, but I knew that bursting into tears because of a dead squirrel on the side of the road was pretty extreme, even for vegetarian me. What was happening to me?!

Angry outbursts were common. I even found myself experiencing the intense emotion of despair, which honestly scared me, as I am a relatively positive person. Again, I did not realize that this was all part of the journey into menopause because no one prepared me AND because I had sustained a serious head injury (and emergency brain surgery) a few years earlier. I thought I was experiencing symptoms of post-traumatic brain injury. (Note: I am dealing with PTBI in other ways, but menopause and TBI have since teased out to be separate issues.)

My primary physician could not answer many of my questions. He just shook his head. "I'm not actually sure about that" was often the answer to my many questions. I smiled, took a deep breath (trying to control one of those knee-jerk reactions!), and reminded him that females make up half the population and that he works with women. I suggested he may want to brush up on his knowledge base in this area.

I also found a new doctor—a woman.

Finally, friends my age clued me in on what was actually happening (hormone shifts from an approaching menopause). As a Generation X-er, I grew up in a time when parents didn't really discuss periods, and "the birds and the bees" was left for schools to deal with through health education. Similarly, no one warned me that perimenopause and beyond would be such a crazy, wild tornado. My menopause coaching evolved so I could survive. I realized I needed to coach myself, and I dove in. My sanity and health were at stake.

Despite all the knowledge I have gained up to this point, I am still learning. I am not an expert, but I have cultivated an understanding of the key focus areas a woman in peri-, mid-, and post-menopause will likely need to focus on to ride out this rite of passage in a holistic and healthy way. Based on my experience and training, here are five key areas for women to focus on for a smoother and more fulfilling transition into menopause. This stage of life should not be overlooked or dismissed—it's important to acknowledge it and gain the skills to navigate it with confidence.

Navigating Menopause:
5 Key Areas to Address for a Healthy Transition

Emotions: Menopause brings up *a lot* of emotions. For me, not having children of my own meant that the possibility of motherhood was forever closed, which stirred up deep grief. It's also a time for closure on other chapters of our lives—acknowledging past traumas, grieving what never was, and accepting what can never be. It is important to allow ourselves to feel these emotions fully.

Francis Weller's "The Five Gates of Grief" explores how important it is to process loss in a world that often ignores deep sorrow. Facing personal loss, unloved parts of ourselves, the suffering of the world, unmet needs, and ancestral grief guide us toward healing and connection. When we create the space to experience these feelings, we can release them and embrace the next phase of our lives with grace, readiness, and excitement about what we can create moving forward.

Body Maintenance: This is about food and fitness, but more importantly, it's about helping women in different phases of menopause turn their food and fitness goals into a reality. Most women already know what they should do but struggle to follow through due to busy schedules, uncertainty about where to start, or fear of change. Life inevitably gets in the way, making it difficult to stay consistent.

That's where coaching comes in—providing strategies, accountability, and personalized support to create lasting change in a way that feels inspiring and sustainable. Menopause coaching focuses on incorporating regular exercise into your life by finding the right routine for both fitness and hormone balance. Additionally, it helps women understand how to eat for nutrition, hormone regulation, weight maintenance, and sustained energy. With practical food formulas, meal planning, and prepping strategies, menopause coaching simplifies the process of nourishing the body while navigating this life transition.

Mindset: Stress management must become a top priority for women navigating all stages of menopause. Due to hormone dysregulation, cortisol can cause extreme stress. Depression, anxiety, frustration, impatience—many of these moods can overshadow a woman's sense of peace and happiness. Not to mention, menopause-specific challenges like night sweats, sleep issues, and sexual health also come into play. Stress management practices, medical approaches (HRT, doctor-supported treatments, etc.), and natural remedies (herbs, supplements, lifestyle shifts) are also explored to support each person's unique journey.

Personal Growth: The phases of menopause symbolize not just the end of one cycle, but the beginning of another. Self-discovery and personal empowerment have the potential to reside in this place, with the excitement of exploring new passions, honoring personal values, and cultivating personal reinvention. This is about redefining identity, finding purpose in midlife, and embracing change with confidence. Goal strategies come into play here, as well as big-picture thinking (how aligned are you to your ideal life, how authentically are you experiencing your journey, and what is your definition of integrity and fulfillment?).

Community: "I feel invisible" is a sentiment I've heard far too often. Menopause can feel like an isolating journey, but it doesn't have to be. Connecting with other women who are experiencing similar changes creates a powerful support network, offering reassurance, wisdom, and encouragement.

Community is where healing happens—through shared stories, collective learning, and the validation of knowing you're not alone. Group coaching provides a space for honest conversations, emotional support, and practical strategies, making the transition into menopause feel more manageable and even empowering. By fostering these connections, we can redefine this phase of life not as something to endure alone, but as an opportunity to grow stronger together.

Final Thoughts

Navigating menopause can feel like an overwhelming journey, but it doesn't have to be something a woman faces alone. By focusing on key areas like emotions, body maintenance, mindset, personal growth, and community, we can turn this phase of life into one of empowerment and transformation. I am thankful for my tumultuous experience through peri, mid, and post-menopause because I had to coach a very special client: myself. Today, I am very grateful that this experience and training as a menopause coach have equipped me to support women through this transition, offering guidance, strategies, and a safe space for healing and connection. I love being part of this incredible journey and sharing this experience with a community of inspiring and powerful women.

One important way my work has evolved since my own peri- and post-menopause journey is through a deeper understanding of the role alcohol plays during this life stage.

As an alcohol-free lifestyle coach, I now support many women navigating perimenopause and post menopause through this lens. What I've witnessed, both personally and professionally, is how alcohol can quietly amplify many of the very symptoms women are struggling with during this transition: disrupted sleep, heightened anxiety, emotional volatility, increased inflammation, weight changes, and depleted coping capacity.

For me, removing alcohol didn't "fix" menopause—but it dramatically improved my ability to cope, regulate my emotions, listen to my body, and make supportive choices. Without alcohol in the picture, everything became clearer: what my body needed, what my nervous system could handle, and what changes were actually helpful versus numbing.

Today, I help women reduce or eliminate alcohol so they can move through peri- and post-menopause with more stability, clarity, and self-trust. This work is not about rigid rules or perfection. It's about creating a lifestyle that supports hormonal shifts rather than working against them, and learning how to navigate stress, emotions, and identity changes without relying on alcohol as a coping tool.

Menopause is a profound rite of passage. Approaching it with awareness, compassion, and an alcohol-free lens can open the door to a steadier, more empowered, and deeply authentic next chapter.

If you're seeking support during this life stage and are curious about navigating peri or post menopause through an alcohol-free lens, I invite you to reach out for a complimentary conversation: layne@laynewhitley.com. Let's explore what your next chapter can look like—clear, grounded, and fully supported.

Layne Whitley, Alcohol-Free and Menopause Coach

www.laynewhitley.com/coaching

From your first period to PMS to Menopause, there have always been herbs and strategies to support the condition your body is in. Symptoms can vary from mild menstrual cramps to debilitating endometriosis pain. All of these issues can be helped with a combination of nutritional support and herbs, though in some cases you may need help from a physician.

No matter what stage of life you're in, I know that having this advice at hand will help you not feel alone on your life journey. Women all go through the same process—all that's different are the details.

The next section is about men. Whether you are one or just know one, it's going to be as important for you to read that section as it is for men to read the one we just finished.

Chapter 28: Herbal Support for Men

Men frequently ask me about two things: **prostate health** and **erectile dysfunction**. Did you know that the two are related?

Testosterone is the main sex hormone in men. It's essential to a man developing "normal" male characteristics, such as body and facial hair, increased muscle tone, size and stature, and other masculine physical characteristics. Moreover, testosterone directly affects muscle size and strength, libido, testicular development, deepening of the voice, and sperm production (Harvard Health Publishing, n.d.). Testosterone levels in men naturally decrease as they age, but there are some all-natural steps you can take to mitigate this.

Having a balanced, healthy diet combined with regular exercise can solve a majority of the health issues men face today. A healthy diet is one through which you're getting all or most of your vitamins, fats, and minerals from whole food sources. At the bare minimum, regular exercise is taking a 30-minute walk every day, but it is much more beneficial to your health if you incorporate some form of strength training, hiking, yoga, or something more strenuous into your exercise routine.

To get started, follow my previously detailed dietary suggestions (though realize, as a man, you may need to eat a higher quantity of meat than women do) and get your butt outdoors on a regular basis. Don't eat highly processed foods, stay away from energy drinks, limit yourself to no more than two cups of coffee a day (ideally consumed before noon), don't drink soda except as an occasional treat, avoid candy, and learn to cook for yourself. According to research, these simple fixes can help you naturally boost your testosterone production by up to 30% (Fisher, 2024).

Herbs you should be familiar with for prostate health:

Stinging nettle *(Urtica dioica)*: Stinging nettle **root** has been taken to treat benign prostatic hyperplasia and helps lower the incidence of prostate cancer. Taking 1200 mg of stinging nettle root daily for at least four months can significantly decrease an enlarged prostate gland. Stinging nettle leaf is also helpful to know (for both men and women), as it helps your body deal with allergies and is an extremely nutritive tonic herb that can be taken daily as a sort of multivitamin. To learn more about stinging nettle, you can watch my short video lesson (linked in the Additional Resources section at the end of the book).

Saw palmetto berry *(Serenoa repens)*: This plant grows as a wild weed in Florida. Saw palmetto blocks both androgen receptors and the action of estrogen in the prostate. You know how I said red clover competes for estrogen and therefore helps balance it in a woman's body? Similarly, saw palmetto competes for both androgenic and estrogenic receptors in the prostate and acts as a tonic. It can help reduce the size of the prostate and make it easier to pee, especially at night. Men need to be taking this for a minimum of two months before they can expect to see results.

Additionally:

Pine pollen *(Pinus spp.)*: The same yellow stuff that covers your car and driveway in springtime is actually the highest source of natural testosterone found in the plant kingdom. You see, pine trees have been around for millions of years. They developed before insects were around to pollinate plants. Therefore, pine trees pollinate each other whenever the wind blows (during pollinating season, typically around April-May). The pollen from the male trees finds the cones on the female trees and pollinates them, fertilizing the next generation of pine trees.

You can take advantage of this by taking pine pollen powder as a part of your daily smoothie or in tincture form as a daily supplement. Pine pollen has been found to have anti-aging effects as well as the ability to increase overall testosterone levels in both men and women (Wolkodoff, 2024).

To be fair, you may still require testosterone supplementation from your doctor if your levels are too low for the plants to provide sufficient help. But in my opinion, it's best to search for a natural solution first and try it out before deciding to go the pharmaceutical route.

Moving on to the other issue men commonly face, there are two potential physical causes of **erectile dysfunction**: circulation problems and nerve damage.

The most common cause is **circulation problems**, which is also why so many men deal with high blood pressure. Cayenne, ginger, ginkgo biloba, and hawthorn berry have been shown to improve circulation; all of these are safe to take in a capsule, smoothie, or tea. Before trying any spice, herb, etc., you need to check that it's safe to take with any medications you're currently on. Remember, I'm not saying, "Just take this herb, and your erectile dysfunction will be cured!" I'm telling you that these herbs are the ones I would research first.

Following the dietary recommendations we cover in this book, along with getting regular exercise, will help you better manage your weight and blood pressure (both of which directly affect your circulation). Additionally, doing so will improve your nutritional intake so that your health issues may be resolved without the addition of any (or many) herbs. When you do use herbs for their medicinal benefits, it can take several weeks or even months of being on an herbal protocol before you start feeling or seeing results, so you must be patient and consistent.

Maca powder may help improve your sexual desire, as it does in women. When you combine an increased sexual desire with adequate levels of testosterone (pine pollen) and sufficient venous circulation (cayenne pepper and hawthorn berry), you have a recipe for a sexual tonic that may be enough to help your penis become ready for action.

Sexual Tonic Recipe

1 Tbsp Maca powder

1 Tbsp Pine pollen powder

1 Tbsp Hawthorn Berry (powdered)

1 Tbsp Ginkgo biloba leaf powder

½ tsp Cayenne pepper powder

Blend powders together and add to a smoothie or coconut milk (something it can be blended into to improve its taste; experiment to find what you like best). Take daily for best results.

If your ED is caused by **nerve damage**, you'll know because you won't be able to feel anything down there. Whether you touch it, try to masturbate, or clean yourself, it will be either completely or partially numb. You may want to look into herbs like St. John's wort (which can help heal nerve damage when applied topically over several weeks). However, making sure you're getting all the nutrients your body needs to heal and rebuild itself should be your top priority.

Men, please remember to wear underwear made of natural fabrics! Cotton, hemp, or wool will let your groin breathe, while synthetic fabrics will trap heat and moisture against your skin for extended periods of time. Natural fabric underwear are also less likely to restrict blood flow and cause hormonal imbalances than their synthetic counterparts (Shafik, 1993). The same goes for any tight pants you own. Make sure they are breathable, do not cut off your circulation, and do not contain any endocrine disruptors. Wearing cotton underpants won't do you much good if your pants are overly tight and made of polyester (plastic).

Lastly, I encourage you to pick up Stephen H. Buhner's books on men's testosterone support to do more in-depth reading on other ways you can support your body naturally. This becomes even more important as you age, with your testosterone decreasing naturally over time. Why not get a head start on learning what you can do about it? When you reach whatever you would deem to be "old age," the familiar adage goes, "If you haven't got your health, then you haven't got anything."

Chapter 29: Low Libido—Men and Women

Most humans enjoy sex. If you don't enjoy sex, there's a reason (whether it be psychological, emotional, or asexuality-related). But when sexual enjoyment feels like a dream hidden behind a curtain, something you used to experience but can't feel anymore, your brain and body suffer. If you're a woman in perimenopause or menopause, or you're a man over the age of 50, you may be more likely to struggle with libido. You can become depressed or lonely over time, especially if you can't derive enjoyment from masturbation anymore.

This is when you want to see what herbs can do to improve your libido! What follows are only a few of the many herbal aphrodisiacs you can try. Remember, aphrodisiacs work differently in each person's body. One person may experience a strong response to a certain aphrodisiac, while someone else may have no response to the same herb (or food).

In addition to herbs, the prevailing wisdom on aphrodisiac foods suggests that both chocolate and oysters are decent libido tonics. In fact, eating a little dark chocolate can help satiate your desire for sex if you're unpartnered or have a partner who is not in the mood. Keep a high-quality, sustainably and ethically sourced chocolate bar hidden in the back of your freezer for when your partner is unavailable but you've got the urge.

Eating a healthy diet and getting ALL the minerals your body needs, along with getting regular, sufficient exercise, will help every single one of you, no matter what stage of life you're in. The previously mentioned factors—as well as sleep quality, stress levels, and hormone balance—all play a large role in maintaining a healthy libido (NHS inform, 2023).

Low libido can be due to a number of causes, including high stress levels, relationship problems, emotional incompatibility with your partner, lack of good hygiene from your partner, nutritional imbalances, or circulation issues due to age. Low testosterone levels can affect both men and women. If you have your hormone levels tested and your blood work comes back with too-low testosterone levels, you will want to take measures to raise it, such as by adding pine pollen to your daily smoothie or taking a strong pine pollen tincture (Wolkodoff, 2024).

Now, on to the herbs:

Maca *(Lepidium meyenii)*: Sometimes referred to as Peruvian ginseng, maca can be easily found in powdered form and added to your daily smoothie. Capsules are also readily available. Maca can be helpful for treating erectile dysfunction in men and for increasing sexual desire in women. I can personally attest to the fact that when I first started adding maca to my smoothies, my libido jumped! Since I've been taking it for a few years now, the novelty has worn off. It also acts as an energy tonic, so if you struggle with low energy, this herb is worth adding to your daily regimen.

Tribulus *(Tribulus terrestris)*: This herb is most often seen as a supplement recommended to help increase testosterone in men, as well as increase their health and stamina. It is a major player in many of the men's sexual health herbal blends I've seen online. Taken daily, it can act as a restorative tonic in older men.

As a warning, here's my secondhand experience with this herb: I suggested tribulus to a very close friend of mine to help him with his libido. After taking it daily for about a week, he developed a bad snoring problem. It was so bad that his partner was leaving the room in the middle of the night to escape his snoring and going to sleep on the sofa! As soon as he stopped taking the tribulus, the snoring subsided. As stated previously, every person responds to every herb differently, with this being one such example.

Damiana *(Turnera diffusa)*: This plant is native to Mexico, thriving in dry, arid regions, so I have never seen it growing in the wild where I live. It has antidepressant effects and is a tonic for stress and low energy, which in turn acts to increase your libido. You can take it as a tea, tincture, or as part of an herbal smoking blend to experience its effects.

Before ending this chapter, I want to cover a few more topics regarding sex. And remember, this is coming from a woman who has been around a while, has had multiple sexual partners (all men), and was married twice. I've also been through a major mental breakdown and years of intensive therapy in order to finally heal my mental health. Having said all that:

If you are not satisfied with your current sex life, there is a reason.

I'm not talking about your partner being bad in bed or not having the right size genitalia. I'm not talking about how one of you wants to do it more often than the other or that you argue about whether to use toys in the bedroom or not. Here, I'm referring to a much more nuanced issue. If you are not being fulfilled physically, mentally, emotionally, and spiritually in your relationship, there's very little chance you'll be fulfilled sexually.

Sex is more than just a physical act. In order to be truly satisfied, you need to find someone who can fulfill your needs in all areas. Otherwise, you're just fucking each other. And fucking gets boring real fast. Physically forcing your body to have an orgasm may give a fleeting sense of pleasure but can leave you feeling empty emotionally and mentally.

When you are with someone who understands you, you both want to please one another, and you are compatible on all levels, that's when sex is truly satisfying. You're not just doing the physical gymnastics of trying new positions, using toys, or allowing your body to be used as a masturbatory tool for the other person. You're connecting on an emotional, mental, and spiritual level. You are satisfying each other's needs in more than just the primal sense of procreation.

This can sound like a dream, a luxury that most people never get to experience. And for many people, it is. But after years of working out how I got so messed up in the first place and healing my emotional, mental, and sexual wounds, I now know that it IS possible to resolve your sexual trauma and find a partner who can fulfill you in other, more mentally satisfying ways.

The trick is knowing where and how to find it.

If you want to start on the path to finding a partner who will satisfy you in ALL areas, I know who can help you learn about all five areas of fulfillment.

I took his class when I was still married to my previous husband, when I had begun to question my sanity and if it was all worth it, and when I was drinking heavily to numb my feelings. This man's class "Is He A Keeper" opened my eyes to how deeply unsatisfied I was in my marriage. If that's not something you're potentially prepared to face, then his services are not for you.

But if you're searching for how to heal yourself in all the ways that matter and find a partner who will fulfill all your needs, look up Bryan Redfield and check out his classes for men and women. They changed everything I thought I knew about relationships and being happy emotionally.

And lastly, a note about sexual partners:

Remember how we have a gut microbiome? We also have a skin microbiome. When we have a romantic partner who we frequently cuddle or have sex with (and most likely live with), we begin to share that microbiome with each other. In some cases, couples who have been together for several years can have a 70% higher chance of developing their partner's chronic physical ailments due to the exchange of their microbiome (Kiecolt-Glaser et al., 2019).

If you are with a partner who does not take care of their body to the best of their ability, both internally and externally, while YOU are doing your best to take good care of yours, you run the risk of developing some of the same physical problems your partner suffers from. You're sharing skin particles, bacteria, fluids, and who knows what else without even thinking about it.

Consider this aspect of a relationship if you are not currently in one. If you have the ability to choose a partner who shares similar health habits and values with you, you are more likely to get along on an emotional level and not do harm to one another on a microscopic, physical level.

As previously mentioned in the Prevention section, it's important to remember that a woman can get bacterial vaginosis from being intimate with a man who does not properly clean his penis. An uncircumcised man can get a yeast infection from a woman who is suffering from one if they have sex before she is cured of it. If a woman with an active cold sore (oral herpes) goes down on a man with her mouth, he will end up with genital herpes (and vice versa) (Centers for Disease Control and Prevention, 2024).

Note: Uncircumcised men are susceptible to yeast infections in and around the penis head under the foreskin if they have sex with a woman who has an active yeast infection. The best treatment for this is to air out the penis head every day by pulling the foreskin back and doubling up on probiotics while avoiding sugary foods for a few days.

These are just a few examples of regular, non-life-threatening problems that you could experience if you aren't mindful of who you're being intimate with and under what circumstances. These issues can arise for various reasons; it is nothing to feel shame over. But if left unchecked, they can cause immense strain between your intimate partner and yourself, resulting in lowered libido. Sexual fulfillment is one of the great joys we experience as part of the human race. It doesn't matter what your age is; if you used to enjoy having sex and you suddenly don't anymore, there's a reason. Discovering whether that reason is physical, mental, emotional, or maybe even spiritual is your next step to better understanding yourself. There are many resources—self-help books, coaches, and natural health practitioners—that can help guide you through your sexual self-discovery.

My suggestion to you is to simply put it out there to the Universe. Right now, say out loud, "Universe, please show me the solution to my libido problem and help me get it back again." This may seem silly, but asserting your intention is often the first step to evoking change. The next thing you know, you're likely to find the right person or product that will help you along on your journey because you set your intention into motion. Remember, it never hurts to ask for help. You've got this!

Chapter 30: Vaginal Infections

The two most common infections a woman must know about are yeast infections and bacterial vaginosis. Fortunately, the most effective treatment for both is very similar.

Yeast infections are fungal in nature, caused by too much candida in the body and especially in the vaginal canal. Symptoms usually include itchiness and redness in and around the vulva and a milky white, chunky discharge reminiscent of cottage cheese. The vulva area and discharge may smell yeasty, almost like sourdough bread, depending on the severity of the infection.

If you have sexual intercourse with someone while you have a yeast infection, you will transfer your discharge onto their member. If your partner has an uncircumcised penis and you have unprotected sex, they will get a yeast infection in and around their foreskin. Then, you will both have a yeast infection. You will both need treatment before you can safely have sex again; otherwise, you will continue to pass the infection back and forth to each other.

I had chronic yeast infections, at least once every other month for over 17 years. Trust me, I know and have tried every remedy known to woman. I found that the only way to resolve the problem completely is by changing your diet and healing your gut. For me, this meant cutting out wheat and drastically minimizing my sugar intake. Even if you only do this temporarily, it will help. Most of the remedies below work best if you abstain from sugary foods and drinks for at least a few days before, during, and after treatment.

Some of the solutions I know, ranked from least to most effective:

Herbal suppository: Take a small piece of aluminum foil and shape it into a little rectangular boat. In a glass bowl, melt 2 tbsp of raw coconut oil. Add 3 drops of lavender essential oil and 3 drops of tea tree essential oil. Stir, then pour into the mold. Set this in your refrigerator for 10 minutes or until fully solidified. Go to your bedroom, lay a towel down, and lie on top of the towel. Remove the coconut oil suppository from the foil and place it up your vaginal canal as far as you can. Remain lying down for at least 15 minutes (the longer, the better). The towel will catch any of the oil that leaks out of you. This can work to help alleviate a very light yeast infection.

(Note: Don't let this suppository sit in your fridge for more than a few hours. Over time, aluminum foil can leach into whatever is wrapped inside it.)

Apple cider vinegar douche: To do this, you will need a douche kit from your local pharmacy. I don't usually recommend a woman EVER douche her vagina, but if you have a yeast infection, this can sometimes kill the fungus. Douche in the shower so everything rinses down the drain. This treatment works best if you catch the infection early or if it isn't severe.

Garlic: Take a clove of raw garlic and peel it. Stab it a few times with a fork or knife to release the juices. Squat down and place it up your vaginal canal as far as you can. If you get it up there high enough, it will sit atop the pubic bone and usually won't fall out. If you move around a lot, it can wiggle its way down and pop out into your underwear. It's not doing any good unless it's inside your vaginal canal. Leave it inside of you for up to two hours. When you want to remove it, just squat down or go to the toilet to pee and push extra hard like you're pooping. It should pop right out. Discard it into the trash.

(Be aware that doing this treatment will cause the inside of your mouth to taste like garlic. I am unsure why.)

Clotrimazole 1% cream: You can buy this over-the-counter at most pharmacies or even on Amazon. They have 3-day or 5-day treatments. It comes with an applicator and a tube of the antifungal cream you will use. You fill the applicator with the cream and insert it into your vagina every night before bed for the number of days the treatment states. After that time, it should have cured your yeast infection.

I used to have clotrimazole prescribed to me so often—before it was available over-the-counter—that I could just call my doctor, tell her my name, say I had a yeast infection again, and the prescription would be waiting on me at the pharmacy within an hour. It works, but I do not recommend you rely on this for years. Change your diet and save your vagina the headache.

(Note: This is NOT the same thing as Monistat, which does not work.)

Bacterial vaginosis is exactly what it sounds like—a bacterial infection/overload inside the vagina. It results in your crotch smelling like pungent fish. BV is often experienced after a woman has had sex with a man several times in one day without them both fully washing in between sessions. It can also be caused by wearing very tight pants, especially ones made of polyester or rayon fabric that don't allow adequate air flow. BV is preventable, and you can treat it with the same methods as preventing it: air, time, and maybe an extra dose of oral probiotics.

The one preventative measure you MUST do every day or night after you shower is air out your crotch. Go sit on your bed and spread your legs wide so air can flow freely in that area. Move the lips of your vulva around if you have to; you want to get this area as dry as possible. Fungus cannot live where it is dry.

Also, make certain you are wearing underwear, leggings, and pants that are made with natural fibers (only) to further encourage breathability of that area. Synthetic fibers are notorious for trapping heat and moisture against the skin, often leaving your underarms, feet, crotch, and other overly warm areas moist for long periods of time. If your crotch can't breathe, it becomes a perfect host for bacteria and yeast to grow and live. Prioritizing natural fibers is ESSENTIAL for promoting breathability and avoiding yeast infections and BV.

If you're a woman, you will inevitably suffer from a vaginal infection at some point in your life; it is only natural. However, if you are suffering from them perpetually, it may be indicative of a greater issue that needs to be addressed. To prevent vaginal infections, return back to the basics: Keep a healthy diet, support your gut health, wash off after having sex, avoid synthetic and overly tight clothing, and allow breathability in your crotch area. By following these suggestions, you should expect to experience fewer vaginal infections over time.

Chapter 31: Urinary Issues

When you encounter urinary issues, it is often one of two things: urinary tract infection or urinary incontinence. Both can cause great discomfort to the affected person and disruption to daily activity. To start, a **urinary tract infection** is an infection of any part of the urinary tract (bladder, kidneys, urethra, etc.). While women experience UTIs at a significantly higher rate, men can suffer from them as well. They are most often caused by bacteria.

In addition to the airing out step discussed in the previous chapter, the one step you must always take to avoid a urinary tract infection is to pee after having sex. This will cleanse the urethra of any bacteria that may have entered it during intercourse. Did you know that urine is sterile? Every time you pee, your urine cleans your urethra out, expelling bacteria the way it was designed to.

One of the most well-known remedies for treating a UTI is cranberry juice. If you try this, make sure you get 100% cranberry juice for this remedy to be most effective. You can drink it straight, diluted with water, or eat raw, fresh cranberries regularly to support your urinary health. I prefer to buy them frozen and add them to my smoothies.

Herbal remedies for urinary tract infections include cleavers, corn silk, juniper berry, and usnea (which all work well in tea form). You don't need to combine all of these. As long as you get at least one of them, it can help alleviate your UTI. I still say that prevention is best, but in worst-case scenarios, I have used a supplement to treat a UTI with great success.

Urinary Incontinence

There are four times in life (outside of an injury or specific disease) someone may have bladder problems:

- As a child, wetting the bed at night
- During pregnancy, when the weight of the baby is pressing on the bladder
- During perimenopause and menopause, when the bladder becomes weaker
- In old age, when the muscles around the bladder naturally begin to deteriorate

As with UTIs, both men and women can suffer from urinary incontinence, especially as they age. For men, urinary incontinence most often accompanies other health issues such as prostate issues, nerve damage, and weakened pelvic floor muscles. For women, it most often occurs following physical changes related to pregnancy and childbirth and during major hormonal shifts (such as during menopause).

For most of these circumstances, I suggest you try corn silk as a tea or tincture. Organic corn silk (*Zea mays*) can strengthen the bladder walls and calm inflammation in the urinary tract. If you are pregnant, cranberry juice and red raspberry leaf tea would be helpful daily tonics for you to try. To learn more about stopping urinary incontinence, you can watch my short video lesson (linked in the Additional Resources section at the end of the book). And to learn more about corn silk, you can watch my short video lesson (also linked at the end of the book).

There are many herbal remedies that can help support your urinary tract, whether you're dealing with infection or incontinence. As with everything else in this book, if the natural methods I suggest here aren't improving your condition or if your symptoms worsen, seek guidance from your doctor. Often, you will need to do your own research to find what combination of herbal support and medical treatment works best for you.

Chapter 32: "Doing a Detox" and Kidney Support

Detoxification is the physiological or medicinal removal of toxic substances from a living organism, including the human body, which is mainly carried out by the liver. Your body has four major organ systems responsible for eliminating toxic buildup in your system. We already talked about your lymphatic system. The other three systems are your kidneys, liver, and skin.

How often should you do a detox to cleanse your body? The answer might surprise you, but in my opinion, almost never. Over the years, I know a lot of experts and companies have claimed that the best way to heal this, that, and the other is by doing a full-body detox. But the truth is that your body has wonderful detoxification systems already in place. All you really need to do is support them.

By supporting your body's natural systems of detoxification and elimination, you prevent the need to go to extremes. Such detox protocols may include—but are not limited to—purchasing and taking a pile of special herbs for a week, consuming only three kinds of juices for a set number of days, drinking the milk from a mountain goat whose name was Susie, or exclusively eating foods that will inevitably make you poop your pants.

MOST of the time, the average person can take more mild, balanced steps to support their organs, allowing detoxification and elimination to occur normally. I'm not going to tell you to forgo a recreational enema or a week-long sweat lodge if that's what you want to do. There are spiritual reasons and some very specific medical reasons that you may decide to ignore my advice and do what you know is right for you. (However, I am writing this book from a more straightforward perspective, offering steps that are generally accessible to the majority of people.)

Your **kidneys** filter your blood, regulate fluid balance, and produce hormones, playing a crucial role in overall health. Additionally, they remove waste products, maintain electrolyte balance, and help control your blood pressure. They are the reason you pee, and if they're working well, they're the reason your pee is the right color. (National Institute of Diabetes and Digestive and Kidney Diseases, 2018)

A simple, inexpensive way to help support your kidneys is to drink a glass of warm water with a wedge of lemon squeezed into it first thing in the morning. This is what I use to swallow the bulk of my vitamins and supplements for the day. If your kidneys are struggling, manifesting in the form of edema or frequent kidney stones, consider drinking a small glass of organic celery juice once or twice daily.

Note: If you're frequently eating foods that are high in oxalates—such as purslane, rhubarb, sorrel, spinach, or Swiss chard—you could end up overworking your kidneys (Bargagli et al., 2020). While these foods are generally good for you, as they're rich in vitamins and minerals, it is best to consume them in moderation to avoid the formation of kidney stones.

Some herbs to research for kidney support:

- Burdock root (*Arctium lappa*)
- Corn silk (*Zea mays*)

- Dandelion leaf (*Taraxacum officinale*)
- Juniper berry (*Juniperus spp.*)
- Stinging nettle seed (*Urtica dioica*)
- Stone breaker (*Chanca piedra*)
- Uva ursi (*Arctostaphylos uva-ursi*)

If you are in an advanced stage of kidney disease or are dealing with the aftermath of a kidney transplant, please be VERY careful which herbs you take and how much you take. Some of the above herbs may not be safe if you have advanced problems (American Kidney Fund, 2024). I have heard very good things about stinging nettle seed in more advanced cases, but you should decide which herbs (if any) are right for you based on professional medical advice and what your research yields.

ALWAYS check with your doctor before attempting to replace any medications with a natural supplement. With herbal support, you want to start with lower doses to see if a given herb helps and slowly work your way up until results can be observed. If you experience no results or experience unpleasant symptoms within two weeks of taking any given herb, stop taking it and allow your body a resting period of a few days before testing another. Whether you try an herb via tea, tincture, or capsule is up to your own preference.

Dandelion leaf may be a particularly good option to consider if you're dealing with edema, which is when your legs and feet are very swollen at the end of the day. A doctor will normally prescribe "water pills" for edema; these can help but can also cause potassium depletion inside the body (Clare et al., 2009). Drinking several cups of dandelion leaf tea every day can help relieve water retention with the added bonus that it replaces any lost potassium since it happens to be high in that mineral.

There are two instances I can think of when you may want to do a detox, with the first being in the form of a **parasite cleanse**. Now, I'm not one of those people jumping on the fad boat of "parasites cause every problem known to man!" But I will admit that it's likely far more people have parasites than we once believed possible in our "developed nation."

I personally do a parasite cleanse once, sometimes twice, every year. But hear me out—I'm a forager! I don't always wash what I forage before I put it in my mouth and eat it. If I'm out in the woods and I see something I want to snack on, it might get wiped on my pants at best before it becomes my mid-foraging snack. It certainly isn't getting a full produce wash treatment. I can guarantee I have eaten slug poop at some point and was none the wiser.

If you're living a lifestyle similar to mine, there's a possibility you share the same risk as I do. (Here, I am not referring to such activities as foraging near dog poop or sewage plants; I am referring to foraging in wild, uncontaminated areas.) I make a parasite cleanse tincture with the fresh green husks of black walnuts (*Juglans nigra*), cloves (*Syzygium aromaticum*), raw garlic (*Allium sativa*), and wormwood (*Artemesia absinthium*). This kills all stages of most parasites in your digestive system. I take a half dropperful of this tincture in a glass of water three times daily with a single activated charcoal capsule once daily to help expel the dead parasite bodies through my poop.

If you are actively seeing worms in your poop, have a super itchy butthole (especially at night), or are losing weight rapidly (while eating normally), please go to your doctor and get tested for parasites. They can give you something much stronger than my herbal cleanse that will kill whatever parasite is inhabiting your body.

The second instance when detoxification may be necessary is when **mold** is found to be present in your body or environment. Exposure to mold is more likely to result in symptoms if you have a mold allergy or sensitivity, asthma or another respiratory condition, hay fever, or an immune condition. It can also affect you more strongly if you are on a medication that suppresses your immune system.

Humans are exposed to mold every single day. Our bodies are built to withstand the normal amounts of mold, bacteria, spores, yeasts, etc. that are floating in the air. Every individual has a different tolerance to the amount of mold their body can handle before they begin showing symptoms, based on their immune system and overall health (Hardin et al., 2003).

However, there are times you may discover you have toxic levels of mold in your home or workplace that are much higher than your body is able to withstand. To help your body detoxify from mold, the best thing you can do is remove yourself from the environment where it is growing and have the space treated. This is an expensive process, but it beats moving. If you believe you may be experiencing mold inside your body, you can get a mycotoxin test online or from your doctor.

If you have mold toxicity, it would be best to stick very closely to the whole foods-based diet outlined in Part One of this book. While treating mold, you should avoid eating fermented foods, aged or moldy cheese, corn, mushrooms, peanuts and peanut butter, grapes, and melons, as they could possibly feed the mold in your body.

Eating plants high in chlorophyll, like algae, chlorella, or spirulina, can further help detox your body of mold. I take the Saluz™ AFA Wild Harvested Blue Green Algae supplement daily, which helps support detoxification as well as gut health. Cilantro, whether you love it or hate it, is also known to help your body detox from mold overgrowth. Avoiding sugar is critical while treating your body for mold. Exercising daily is equally as important to support removal of toxins through your lymphatic system.

While your kidneys generally do a great job on their own at filtering and excreting liquid toxins from your body, there are a few instances when they may need some extra help. If you are drinking plenty of water and taking measures to support your kidneys and still end up developing kidney stones or a kidney infection, you should assess your diet and try to deduce the cause. Generally, by following a whole foods-based diet and drinking enough water, you're covering the major bases in supporting your kidneys.

Chapter 33: Liver, Gallbladder, and Pancreas Support

The three organs covered in this chapter are all part of your digestive system. Your liver produces bile, which helps you digest and process fats in your food. Your gallbladder decides when to release that bile. Your pancreas releases enzymes that aid your body's digestion. Without them all working as a cohesive team, your digestive tract cannot function at its best. If you have part of your liver removed or if part of it dies, it can regenerate itself. But if you have one of the other two organs removed, you will need to take steps to support your body through other means, such as through supplementation.

Your liver is responsible for filtering toxins out of your blood, such as drugs (pharmaceuticals, over-the-counter, and illicit substances), alcohol, chemicals in your food, and any other harmful substances (Johns Hopkins Medicine, 2025b). It produces bile, which helps your body absorb and digest fats. It also stores vitamins and minerals, regulates blood clotting, and removes bacteria from your bloodstream. You can easily support your liver by eating apples, berries, beets, dark leafy greens, high-fiber cruciferous vegetables, and fish.

I am taking this chapter as an opportunity to explain why everyone is warning you to not take St. John's Wort internally (tea, tincture, capsule.) The reason is **not** that St. John's Wort (*Hypericum perforatum*) interacts poorly with every medication.

The reason is that this herb actually improves the functioning of your liver SO much that it will push your medication through your system faster than it was meant to go, making your medication either not work very well or not work at all. It's best to research or ask your doctor before trying this herb as an internal supplement.

If you're not on any pharmaceutical medication, St. John's Wort could potentially be helpful in supporting detoxification of your liver in certain conditions. As always, do your research before trying it. It's worth noting that when applying this herb externally as an infused oil, the actions are quite different, as referenced in other chapters.

The health and functioning of your liver is of critical importance to your hormone health, especially as a woman. Many women who repeatedly wake up in the middle of the night between 1 am and 3 am, especially if they're going through perimenopause, have a liver that could use support. Consider re-evaluating your relationship with alcohol and start taking measures to support your liver. I personally like taking a liver support supplement and take 1-2 before bed every night.

Some common herbs and root vegetables that help support liver (and gallbladder) function:

- Artichoke leaf (*Cynara scolymus*)
- Beets (*Beta vulgaris*)
- Burdock root (*Arctium lappa*)
- Dandelion root (*Taraxacum officinale*)
- Milk thistle seed (*Silybum marianum*)
- Yellow dock root (*Rumex crispus*)

Excessive alcohol or drug consumption can put stress on your liver (yes, this even includes "safe" drugs like Tylenol). I thank the universe every day that I never got into doing drugs, but I will admit that I was an alcoholic for years. My tactic back then, when I first started learning herbalism, was to only drink wine (because it's supposedly healthier) and to take liver support capsules every morning that I woke up with a hangover. I would take liver-supporting herbs every time I had more than one drink, which was often, and say to myself, "I'm practicing herbalism!" All the while, I was doing damage to my liver, one of the body's most critical organ systems.

On the bright side, eating a plant-based diet—meaning you're eating more fruits and vegetables than any other food group, not that you stop eating meat—and getting adequate exercise are the two main steps to maintaining healthy liver function once you have given up drinking and taking drugs.

Is that too hard? It is for most people. Even I still like to occasionally *taste* something alcoholic now and then. But now it's mainly for the flavor rather than the buzz. Here's the truth: There's a big difference between the people who have a glass of wine once every few months versus the folks who drink a few bottles of wine, a case of beer, a handle of rum, etc., every week.

Making permanent lifestyle changes is hard. If you stopped drinking alcohol, would you still have something to do with your time? Would you still have friends? It's important that you find things that are fulfilling to you outside of drinking, smoking, etc. When you're quitting these habits, you will be alone with your thoughts since you won't have alcohol or drugs to fill your time and attention. If you are able to learn how to be happy spending time by yourself, then you will be able to stop using substances to quiet your thoughts, numb your pain, or continue fitting in with your friend group.

You may lose friends once you stop drinking, smoking, or whatever your shared behavior was, but what is truly important is that you will be able to like, love, and accept yourself. Do what's important for YOU. You have this life to live right here, right now, and you will always be answering to yourself in the end.

If you are struggling with addictive behaviors that are keeping you from achieving your health goals, please read Chapter Thirty-Eight. There, you will read about the importance of developing coping skills that will help you not succumb to old, harmful patterns. I also offer a "How to Quit Smoking Complete System" that instructs you on how to stop drinking alcohol as well.

Your **gallbladder** is an essential part of your digestive system. I don't care if your doctor told you that you would be fine without it. That's kind of like saying you'd be fine with only one eye. Yeah, it's true, but your body was meant to have two, and the loss of one drastically impacts how your vision works. It's the same with your gallbladder, acting as a part of your digestive system. It's basically the holding tank for the bile that your liver produces. It is responsible for releasing bile in your body every time you eat fatty or oily foods, which is pretty important if you want to be able to eat and digest meat.

Some fat is good for you! But if you have a problem with your gallbladder, or you have unfortunately had to have it removed, you still need a way to get bile into your digestive tract to help aid your digestion. Any time you are eating meat or any meal with fat in it, I suggest you take ox bile. You can buy this in capsule form and take one with every meal.

Eating fruits and vegetables puts the least amount of strain on your gallbladder. If you are experiencing gallbladder problems, doing a one-week-long juice cleanse (during which time you only drink fruit/vegetable juices and/or smoothies the entire week), plus taking a few select herbs, can help reset your gallbladder. It's not my definition of fun, but if you're facing the possibility of losing your gallbladder, it may be worth a try.

Gallbladder Cleanse Smoothie

1 cup of mixed fruit (apple, blueberries, cherries, cranberries, mango, orange, pineapple, raspberries, strawberries, etc.)

1 cup of mixed vegetables (beets, celery, cucumber, kale, radishes, spinach, wild-foraged greens, etc.)

3/4 cup 100% fruit juice or coconut water (containing no added sugar)

1-2 Tbsp hemp seed or hemp protein powder

2 Tbsp raw apple cider vinegar

1 Tbsp lemon juice

1 tsp powdered milk thistle seed

Instructions:

Put all ingredients in your blender and blend until smooth. If the flavor is not sweet enough for you, add 1 Tbsp raw honey and blend again. This smoothie can help support your gallbladder, liver, and pancreas by having it a few times a week.

Another herbal hack you can utilize is to take a dropperful of **herbal bitters** prior to eating every meal. What are bitters? Herbal bitters are more than just a bitter-tasting spring plant. They help prime your liver and gallbladder to excrete a little extra bile to aid digestion and cleanse your body of all the heavy buildup that's been stagnating inside you. When you're feeling sluggish, what you often need are some bitter salad greens and a good long poop.

Think about this: You've been stuck indoors most of the winter, keeping warm with lots of hot and hearty chowders, soups, root vegetables, and cocoa. You haven't been working outdoors or going out much aside from an occasional walk, and your body is feeling flimsy and heavy. The first warm, sunny day of spring arrives, and what do you crave? A salad!

This is the tale of our ancestors since time immemorial. After a long winter of surviving the dark, cold season, our bodies crave fresh greens, most of which are somewhat bitter. It's the same reason people eat a salad at the beginning of every fancy meal: The bitter greens prepare your body to digest the main dish, which often includes fats and meats.

If you are unable to forage any bittercress, chicory leaf, dandelion greens, endive, mugwort, or other bitter greens, you can buy bitters ready-made or order the dried ingredients online to make some herbal bitters yourself. Bitters are more than just a flavoring for alcoholic beverages. They're ancient herbal medicine. Experiment with combining different herbs and spices to create more complex flavors as you get better at crafting your own recipes.

Simple Bitters Recipe

6 cardamom pods

1 thumb of fresh ginger, sliced or grated

1 peel and white pith from a small organic orange, chopped (do not add the orange)

¼ cup dandelion root, washed and chopped

1 Tbsp mugwort or wormwood

(Optional: 2 Tbsp yellow dock root, washed and chopped)

1½ cups vodka

Instructions:

Mix all dry ingredients into a pint or quart glass jar. Pour alcohol in and shake well. Allow it to sit on your countertop out of direct sunlight for 2-4 weeks, shaking it occasionally. Then, strain out the solids and bottle your bitters. Take 1 dropperful before each meal. For further instruction, you can watch my herbal bitters recipe video (linked in the Additional Resources section at the end of the book).

The final organ we will cover in this chapter is your **pancreas**. It has two main responsibilities: 1) it produces hormones that help regulate blood sugar in your body, and 2) it produces enzymes to aid in overall digestion.

Eating a wide and varied diet that includes fats and meats (in moderation) along with plenty of plant-based foods is critical to maintaining pancreatic health. Taking ginger or turmeric can help aid digestion and inflammation inside the gut if you're dealing with pain that stems from a compromised pancreas. To learn more about pancreatic care, I would refer you to the web article "The Ins and Outs of Holistic Nutrition for Pancreatic Health."

Your liver, gallbladder, and pancreas are essential to the proper and optimal functioning of your digestive tract. And as you're already aware from previous discussions herein, your digestive tract is responsible for absorbing and processing the nutrients from the foods you eat. You want to do everything you can to support these organs while also abstaining from activities that would do them harm.

My hope is that you are in tune with your body—enough to notice when something is wrong so you can go to the doctor to have it checked out. Once you know what the problem is, you can choose what solution is best for you. Surgery is often the option that a doctor will suggest, but it's not always the option you need to take. It's important that you utilize your doctor for having tests done and getting an accurate diagnosis, after which point you can decide how to proceed based on what you feel is right for your body.

Chapter 34: High Blood Pressure and Cholesterol

High blood pressure, or hypertension, happens when the force of the blood moving through your veins and arteries is too high, causing it to press against the walls of your veins. It is often caused by a combination of factors, including genetic predisposition, but is often exacerbated by poor diet, lack of exercise, smoking, and stress.

Stress is one of the worst culprits, as it is a problem many of us cannot avoid, whether we consider ourselves healthy or not. The good news is that there are some simple things you can do to reduce stress and alter your lifestyle, resulting in lowered blood pressure. They are as follows:

1. **Reduce your salt intake**. Simply saying no to your favorite potato chips and choosing lower-sodium options of the foods you buy will help a great deal, as will cooking most of your meals at home, where you can control how much salt you add.

2. **Take a walk every day**. Simple movement like walking does your body more good than you can imagine! Either try to fit in a 30-minute walk after you get home or see if you can walk for just ten minutes after breakfast, lunch, and dinner. Or perhaps you can get in a two-hour-long hike a couple of days each week. Making sure you move your body will pump lymph through your system, help

you maintain a healthy body weight, and naturally reduce your blood pressure after several weeks of doing so regularly. The great news is that exercise also releases endorphins that lower your stress levels.

3. **If you smoke, quit**. I'm not going to belittle you by telling you all the reasons this is a good idea. If you want help, you can get my Complete Stop Smoking System. It also has instructions to help you quit drinking alcohol and is the same method I used to finally end my alcohol addiction. Once you feel what it's like to be truly healthy and you have the tools to maintain your stress levels without addictive substances, you'll never want to go back.
4. **Eat more fiber**! Again, following the dietary recommendations given in Part One of the book will help you a great deal. If you must have grains, choose oatmeal or buckwheat porridge in the morning. Add some cinnamon, maple syrup, and raisins. I promise you it tastes better than the Quaker Oatmeal packets you grew up on. To get fiber, beans are a great choice, as are just about any fruit or vegetable. Snack on an apple with peanut or almond butter every day, and you'll be surprised how satisfied you feel afterward.
5. **Do your research**. *The Great Cholesterol Myth* is a great read and will give you insight as to why cholesterol has been demonized and why common problems like high stress and too much sugar in your diet are truly to blame for heart disease (Bowden & Sinatra, 2020).
6. **Motherwort** (*Leonurus cardiaca*) is one of the very best herbs for reducing blood pressure. It also has a relaxing

effect on your mind and body. It's most commonly taken as a stress-relief herb. It works best as a tincture, as it is extremely bitter. A general dose is a half dropperful of tincture to start with, taken several times a day.

The main concern here is that if you take motherwort multiple times a day, it's not really any different than you taking a blood pressure drug. It's addressing the symptom rather than the problem. You can keep a bottle of motherwort tincture on hand as a sort of natural rescue remedy for times your blood pressure gets too high, but please don't solely rely on this herb without taking any of the aforementioned steps. Use caution when trying this herb if you are already taking medication to lower your blood pressure, as they can interact.

7. **Lower your stress**. High stress causes high blood pressure. Chapter Thirty-Eight covers methods and herbs that help relieve stress. If drinking a cup of tulsi tea every four hours keeps you out of the hospital ward, isn't it worth the fuss?

Take care of yourself. At the end of the day, you're the only one who can.

General Heart Health

Let's keep it simple: diet and exercise. Changing the way you eat and increasing your intake of fruits and vegetables will help your heart health. Exercising just 30 minutes a day will reduce your risk of cardiac issues (and cardiovascular disease mortality) by 28% to 38% (Berg, 2024). However, it takes time to see the effects of these lifestyle changes.

If you're concerned about your heart, look up hawthorn berry and hawthorn flower. Please do sufficient research if you're already taking heart medication. If there are no interactions between your medication and hawthorn, it's possible this herb, taken as a capsule or tincture, could help protect your heart.

Hawthorn berry (*Crataegus spp.*) preparations, including capsules, teas, and tinctures, improve circulation in the heart as well as improve its oxygen uptake. Further, hawthorn berry can dilate blood vessels to reduce strain on the heart and can improve a cardiac patient's tolerance to exercise when taken in conjunction with a diuretic (such as cleavers or dandelion leaf). Hawthorn berry helps reduce stress and, like rose, soothes a grieving heart. The berries are highly nutritious and are often made into jams and jellies.

Hawthorn flowers (*Crataegus spp.*) are a safe herb to incorporate into your daily regime and can be made into a lovely tea or elixir for their mild cardioprotective properties. They have been studied and proven to improve heart function and reduce the incidence of heart failure (Tassell et al., 2010). The flowers' essence helps work on your mind and spirit energetically; it "channels and purifies the potent will forces of the heart so they become a vehicle of even greater love, compassion, and service on behalf of others" (Kaminski, 2016).

Cayenne pepper (*Capsicum annuum*) can help thin your blood when taken daily in a smoothie or in your food. It may help improve blood flow through your arteries and veins, addressing venous insufficiency and strengthening your arteries (Johns Hopkins Medicine, 2023).

Again, if you're on any kind of heart medication, please consult your doctor before starting a new herbal regimen.

A strong heart is a healthy heart! If you have an office job, try to get up and move around for just 30-60 seconds every 20 minutes or so. This reminds your heart that it needs to keep working and helps you break up the monotony of your day. Any practice that helps activate your heart (like looking at and smelling roses, thinking about your partner or your crush, etc.) will give your heart a happy little push throughout the day and help you maintain healthy blood flow throughout your body.

Chapter 35: Thyroid Problems

Your thyroid is a gland located at the base of your throat that hugs your esophagus. It's responsible for creating most of the hormones your body uses to function. It plays a major role in the growth, development, and health of the human body as well as directly affecting its metabolism (Institute for Quality and Efficiency in Health Care, 2024). It's an essential part of your body's mechanics, despite what doctors may tell you about being able to live without it.

When your thyroid is removed, either fully or partially, you lose the hormonal regulation that your thyroid is meant to provide—regulating your mood, skin health, hair oil production, hunger, and sleep. From that point on, you'll need medication to replace the hormones your thyroid would have produced in order for your body's many systems to continue functioning properly.

Other than the loss of one's thyroid, there are two common problems people have that are related to their thyroid gland—either it's not working well enough or it's working too well. We'll address these issues now.

Hypothyroidism is when your thyroid levels are too low and your body feels sluggish. Those experiencing hypothyroidism are susceptible to constipation and fatigue, are at an increased risk of high cortisol and weight gain, and are frequently cold or have dry skin.

My favorite way to naturally support hypothyroidism is with herbs such as gotu kola (*Centella asiatica*) and tulsi (*Ocimum tenuiflorum*), which both support mood regulation. Additionally, I recommend following a gluten-free, cane sugar-free diet that's rich in whole foods. You can also consider supplementing with desiccated pig thyroid capsules, kelp or seaweed powder, and chlorophyll. I absolutely love the Saluz™ AFA Wild Harvested Blue Green Algae supplement, which I take daily for its many health benefits.

Black walnut (*Juglans nigra*) hull tincture can also be helpful in supporting hypothyroidism, mainly because it helps regulate gut dysbiosis. Eating beef liver weekly or taking a good-quality beef liver supplement can go a long way toward balancing your hormones, as it provides a host of the necessary minerals your body does not get from the other foods you eat. These liver-specific minerals are required for the movement of iron and vitamins in your body. Just make sure you eat your liver with onions, as onions are a source of vitamin C, which is crucial for iron's absorption into your bloodstream.

What follows is an adrenal cocktail that can help give you a quick boost of energy if your body has been feeling sluggish or stress has been keeping you down. Take this during your mid-morning or mid-afternoon slump instead of having another cup of coffee. To see how I make it, you can watch my video tutorial (linked in the Additional Resources section at the end of the book).

Hypothyroid Low Energy Quick Fix Recipe

½ cup fresh orange juice with pulp (OR a handful of fresh rose hips would be an excellent herbal version with a much lower sugar content)

½ cup pure coconut water (sugar-free)

¼ tsp cream of tartar

Pinch of sea salt

Instructions:

Add all ingredients to a blender and pulse for ~15 seconds. That's it! Serve and enjoy.

Hyperthyroidism is less common than hypothyroidism and is essentially the opposite; it is when your thyroid levels are too high. Your body may feel wired or shaky and burn fat more quickly, causing you to become quite thin or gaunt. Additionally, you may have trouble tolerating heat, trouble sleeping, and trouble in the bathroom, experiencing more frequent than usual bowel movements.

Methods I have researched to support this condition include healing the gut via extensive use of probiotics, eating a gluten-free diet, and taking an herbal tea or tincture made with bugleweed (*Lycopus europaeus*) and lemon balm (*Melissa officinalis*). Both of these herbs grow readily and abundantly here in the North, and you only have to plant them once before they will likely spread further into your yard than you ever expected them to. If you have hyperthyroidism, go easy on the kelp or iodine supplements, as too much iodine can exacerbate the condition.

Note: The previously detailed adrenal cocktail won't hurt you if you want to try it, but you may not need it. If anything, you may consider trying milky oats, peach leaf, skullcap, tulsi, or other calming herbs to help you relax. You can take these calming herbs in both tea and tincture form to see which method works best for your body.

Now that we've covered the differences between hypothyroidism and hyperthyroidism, I want to tell you where I would start my thyroid research if I were you: by Googling "American Herbalists Guild Hypothyroid." What comes up is a paper (in downloadable PDF format), written by Cara O'Neal, titled "Herbal and Nutritional Therapeutics for Autoimmune Hypothyroidism." You should print this paper out so you can quickly and conveniently reference it anytime you need to.

As with all things, I took what I found to be useful from the reading and left the rest. The parts of the paper I found useful were the suggestions to take kelp for its iodine, to eat more brassicas (broccoli, cabbage, collards, and kale), and to stop eating wheat (2017). Simply taking these steps, if you still have your thyroid gland, should support your health and transform your negative thyroid symptoms immensely.

The parts of the paper that don't resonate with me are less of a disagreement and more of a preference. Some of the herbal support it recommends are adaptogenic herbs. While adaptogens can be helpful in some cases, I feel that your first step in addressing any thyroid or hormone problem ought to be dietary rather than herbal. You don't *just* want to reduce or cover up your symptoms; you want to resolve the source so they cease completely. (Please refer to Chapter Thirty-Seven for a more in-depth discussion on adaptogens.)

To close the chapter, I am going to tell you my story: I was working two part-time jobs in 2021 along with growing my farm business. As the summer progressed, I noticed that almost every time I swallowed or turned my head to the right, I could feel a lump in my throat. It was as if something was tugging on my Adam's apple area any time I turned. It was uncomfortable, and after it had not gone away after four months, I finally decided I needed to go to the doctor to have it checked out. (This was in September.)

I went to my primary care doctor, and she felt my throat. She said she couldn't feel anything, but I suggested that maybe it was an issue with my thyroid gland. At the time, when I felt my throat, I could feel a small lump in the area to the left of my voice box (right around the middle of my throat).

Back then, I thought the thyroid sat much higher and was smaller than it actually is. You can Google where your thyroid sits if you're unsure, like I was. It's located at the base of your throat and wraps around your esophagus, a little above the collarbone area. Although I was mistaken in my anatomical memory, the doctor agreed that it needed to be checked and sent me for an ultrasound of my thyroid.

When the appointment time came, I went in for the scan. An ultrasound is not scary and doesn't take very long, plus the technician isn't allowed to tell you what they do or don't see. They legally have to wait for the doctor to interpret the results and give you the diagnosis. I got the scan finished and went home.

A few days later, I was working at my farm job, weeding a bed of green beans, when my phone rang. I answered it and was met with one of the most frightening calls you can ever receive from a physician: "We found a lump, and we want to send you in for a biopsy."

I made the appointment, of course. When I got off the phone, my hands were shaking. My boss, the farm owner, was nearby working in the gardens as well, and I told her what had just happened. She could see that I was pretty shaken up, but she assured me that it was just a biopsy and I was probably fine.

As a precaution, I began taking turkey tail tincture every day to help boost my body's ability to fight cancer. It turns out that most mushrooms have cancer-fighting properties, so I've been taking turkey tail along with several other mushrooms in double-extracted tincture form ever since. To this day, if anyone asks me what to do to help your body fight cancer, whether that's preventive or you are actively battling it, my first thought goes to mushrooms.

I went in for the biopsy a couple of weeks after that call. I spent about an hour with my head tilted back, staring at the ceiling and the wall behind me while a doctor stuck a long needle into my neck. A week later, I was told that I needed to make an appointment to visit with an endocrinologist and a surgeon. I went to every appointment alone.

The endocrinologist told me that the lump they found was about the size of a pea and had a 50% chance of being cancerous. She was surprised and astounded that I was so in tune with my body and able to feel the change. She said that under a normal, yearly checkup schedule, doctors would not have discovered the lump on my thyroid for at least another 3 to 5 years.

The endocrinologist said that while it was ultimately my choice, her professional recommendation was that I have my thyroid removed. I was told that it is impossible to only remove a lump from the thyroid gland because there is such a strong blood supply going through it that I would inevitably bleed to death if they tried. I had the choice of getting a total or partial thyroidectomy.

They suggested I get the whole thing removed "as a precaution," but as the lump was only a concern on the left half of my thyroid, I insisted that they only remove that half. I was adamant. When I consulted with the surgeon himself, I told him to his face that unless he opens me up and unexpectedly finds a whole bunch of cancer all over the place that they didn't know was there, I had better damned well wake up with the good half of my thyroid gland intact.

He agreed. On December 10th, 2021, I went in for surgery. I was still living with my second husband at the time. Thankfully, he took me to the hospital and was there to take me back home after the surgery was over.

After I woke from the operation, the surgeon came in to talk with me. He said it was very interesting when he was operating because as he was removing the left half of my thyroid, he saw the lump of cancer. It had attached itself to some of the muscle tissue on the left side of my neck, explaining why I had felt a "lump" in my throat all that time. The cancer was pulling on my neck muscle every time I turned my head, letting me know it was there.

He thought surely the cancer would have spread into the muscle tissue. But after they tested the lump, cancer was ONLY in the lump itself. Nothing cancerous had spread to anywhere else in my body. I know I was being taken care of. You can call it God, Goddess, Higher Self, Inner Being, the Universe, or whatever you want. But something was looking out for me.

The following month after my scar had healed, I was started on a medication to help normalize my body's TSH (thyroid-stimulating hormone) levels now that half my thyroid was gone. I have two very tiny lumps on the remaining half of my thyroid that the doctor wants to monitor to make sure they don't get larger and potentially develop into cancer as well. If I don't take the medication, the remaining half of my thyroid will grow larger to compensate for the missing half, thus causing those two small lumps to grow as well. This could potentially lead them to turn into cancer, which is what my doctor and I want to avoid.

However, I did not want to put any synthetic medication into my body. I asked my endocrinologist whether there was any natural alternative to the synthetic medication I had been prescribed. She sighed—she had already had enough conversations with me by that time to know that not only was I an herbalist, but I was also keenly aware of how my body worked—and told me that there was ONE natural medication for thyroid help.

I was put on NP Thyroid, also known as Armour Thyroid. It took an entire year to get the dosage just right, which was no easy feat because the medication only comes in 15 mg or 30 mg doses. But we eventually got it right, and I've only had to increase my dose once since then. When you first start taking it, you get a distinct pig taste (like pork) in the back of your throat. It's not pleasant, but it's not the worst thing I've ever ingested. At this point, I don't even notice it anymore.

I did ask my doctor whether it would be possible to simply take desiccated pig thyroid capsules instead of my prescription, in case there came a time I could no longer get my prescription. She said that while technically it is the same thing, the dose in each individual capsule of over-the-counter pig thyroid is both inconsistent and unregulated. Therefore, it would be virtually impossible to get the dosage right.

For women specifically: During the year-long process it took me to figure out just the right dosage of my NP Thyroid medication, my doctor asked me to try the synthetic stuff, Synthroid. I was taking 25 mg a day, and within 24 hours of taking the first capsule, I could feel that something in my body was "off." In fact, by the second day, I had an unusual, smelly vaginal discharge for no apparent reason. That night, I stopped taking the Synthroid and went back to taking NP Thyroid. My symptoms were gone in less than 12 hours. My point being, don't blindly trust synthetic medications just because they're what your doctor prescribes you; only take them if you have no other choice.

The interesting thing is that I have taken rather good care of my body for the last 14 years or so, yet I still ended up with thyroid cancer. Part of this can be explained by the fact that I know my uncle needed his thyroid removed years ago due to a goiter problem. I knew my grandmother had thyroid issues in her old age too.

There is also a much higher prevalence of thyroid cancer in the Northeastern United States. After talking with my endocrinologist about this, our best guess is that the incredible amount of pollution in this area left over from the Industrial Revolution and the numerous toxins leaching into the environment from the thousands of long-dead factories are likely to blame. The Northeast is riddled with the remains of brick factory buildings, most of which are sitting on a veritable toxic dump of chemical runoff from what they used to power factories with in the 19th century. I've not done extensive research on the correlation between the Northeast and thyroid cancer; it's just my hunch.

I was told that because I only have half my thyroid, I should not be supporting it and encouraging it to grow by giving it kelp or other iodine-containing supplements. I was disappointed at hearing this, as I had gotten used to adding a small amount of kelp powder to my dinner every night (it's highly nutritious and tastes a bit salty). However, I noticed that when I stopped taking kelp powder completely, within about six months, the number of cherry angiomas on my skin increased by a LOT. For this reason, I went back to adding ¼ tsp of kelp powder to my daily smoothie, and the angiomas went back to their normal rate of occurrence, occasionally showing up on my body rather than wildly proliferating.

Thyroid problems are more common than you may think, especially in women. If you do encounter them at some point in your life, don't be discouraged! As we have covered in this chapter, there are several ways you can support your thyroid health without needing to go on synthetic medication and be at the mercy of Big Pharma for the rest of your life.

Whether you're experiencing hypothyroidism or hyperthyroidism, a combination of the right nutrition and herbal support is your key to managing the worst of your symptoms. As with the rest of your body-machine, keeping everything in tune and working as a cohesive whole will help you resolve most common health problems on your own.

Chapter 36: Managing Your Weight

Losing weight is not always just calories in, calories out. Having a healthy, functioning gut microbiome that's helping you digest whole foods full of complex carbohydrates, essential fatty acids, and plenty of fiber is the most important key to maintaining a healthy weight.

If you are currently struggling with an eating disorder, please seek professional help from a doctor or nutritionist. Eating disorders often have long-lasting effects, causing damage to multiple parts of your body. They are NEVER a good method for losing (or gaining) weight. You must heal mentally and emotionally from disordered eating before you can expect to be mentally capable of losing (or gaining) the weight you need to be healthy.

Simply cutting (or significantly reducing) cane sugar, soda, wheat, and highly processed foods like cake, cookies, TV dinners, etc. from your diet will cause you to start shedding pounds. Just don't switch from buying Chips Ahoy to buying gluten-free Chips Ahoy. It's just as bad for your blood sugar, trust me.

Do you think I never eat cookies or candy? I do. Sugar is a trap that we all fall into occasionally. The difference is that I am strategic about what I buy. I'm a label-reading fanatic. Before I healed my cane sugar allergy, I was severely limited by what I could and couldn't eat. In all honesty, I am still very careful when deciding what sugar-containing foods I eat. Most of the time, when I want a sweet treat, I bake it myself at home so I know exactly what is going into it.

If you currently drink a lot of soda, do I have the hack for you! Switch to plain seltzer or buy a seltzer maker. It pumps carbonation into your regular water, so you get all the bubbles with none of the sugar. You can buy syrup packets to flavor your drink, but I forego this step to avoid the extra sugar. Instead, I like to squeeze a lime wedge (yes, from an actual lime) into the bottom of my glass and fill it with plain seltzer. This is DELICIOUS and fulfills my desire to drink something other than plain water or tea.

I'm not a fitness professional, personal trainer, or even particularly muscularly toned. I am not an expert in helping people lose weight. From my observations, men seem to be able to drop a hundred pounds just by changing their diet. Women, on the other hand, have a lot more going on in terms of their hormones, which affects our weight just as much as diet and exercise do (Blaak, 2001).

I'm not overweight, but I have a bit of belly fat that is mostly related to my high cortisol levels, causing my body to hold onto the extra pounds because it thinks I'm about to go into a famine state. That's right, depending on the time of year and how I'm feeling, the lady you're getting health advice from deals with "cortisol belly."

I'm telling you this because it happens to the best of us. And it can be depressing! When you go from feeling great in a swimsuit at the beach to six months later pinching your fat roll when you sit down and wondering where the hell it came from, it doesn't feel good. But the good news is that it's most likely subcutaneous fat, which is the kind that's easiest to get rid of.

If that doesn't make sense, let me explain: Women naturally have a higher body fat percentage than men. Our society here in the United States has only been given access to ample calorie sources for approximately the past 100 years (Morrison et al., 2010; Veit, 2018). Before then, our bodies were subject to periods of starvation and periods of plenty. Our bodies naturally carry excess fat around the middle because that's the ideal place to store it when we think we will be facing a period of famine. Most Western cultures are used to food being scarcer from January through March because the world around us is covered in ice and snow. Only in very modern times have we been able to go to the grocery store and buy whatever we want at any time of year.

Women's bodies evolved the ability to retain extra fat around the middle, not only so we could survive, but so our children could survive. If you were a pregnant woman 3,000 years ago and your village experienced a period of famine, you would have a higher chance of surviving (and your baby surviving) if you carried some extra fat on your body. Science is still in debate as to exactly why it tends to pool on the hips and thighs, but fat distribution is actually different across different cultures and genetic regions. Either way, your body is telling you to be prepared in case your food supply runs out while you're lamenting that you won't look thin in a swimsuit this year.

Typically, I gain a little fat back in the wintertime that I may have lost in the warmer seasons. This is partly because I'm indoors most of the time, not getting exercise, and partly because of the vitamin D deficiency that inevitably occurs between February and March. After no ultraviolet sunlight reaches my skin for an extended period of time, my body's vitamin D stores become depleted. During the winter, lack of sun results in seasonal affective disorder for many people, which is basically your sun-deprived body succumbing to vitamin deficiency depression.

I want you to accept that your weight will most likely fluctuate throughout your adult life and that it's OKAY. This is perfectly normal! Do not stress about five pounds. You can lose five or ten pounds easily once the weather warms up and the sun is out.

While mild weight fluctuation and subcutaneous fat are typically harmless, **visceral fat**, the kind of fat that builds up around your internal organs, can be especially dangerous to your health and more difficult to lose. How can you tell the difference? If you can pinch the fat and skin of your waist in your fingers and hold it, then you have **subcutaneous fat**. If, however, your belly is large but feels hard to the touch (think of a middle-aged man with a beer gut), then you most likely have fat built up around your internal organs. Losing this type of fat requires strict adherence to a diet and an exercise routine that is specific to your needs. If you are overweight but most of the fat on your body is not the "pinchable" kind, I would recommend you seek help from a fitness trainer.

Intermittent fasting, the practice of eating during a certain window of time (such as eating between 10 am and 6 pm daily) and only drinking water or tea during your fasting window, may be a good method to try if you're looking to lose weight and reduce inflammation. By eating during a certain window of time and fasting for the rest of the time, you're following an eating-fasting cycle much like our ancestors did, which works with many people's primitive natural rhythm.

IF guidelines are based on sex and weight, so you will need to research what is suitable for you based on these factors (Johns Hopkins Medicine, 2021). It is best to consult with a doctor if you are currently dealing with any health conditions or if you are on any kind of medication. While doing IF, you still need to make sure you're getting a healthy balance of the right foods and meeting your daily caloric needs. There are many different IF variations, which you can learn about in the web article "6 ways to do intermittent fasting."

Finally, eating sufficient fiber, both soluble and insoluble, is critical for weight loss. Fiber intake can increase the efficiency of a "calories in, calories out" style weight loss plan because it binds to cholesterol and helps remove it from the body (Jenko Pražnikar et al., 2023). As covered in Chapter Five, naturally occurring sugar-rich foods are always accompanied by a source of fiber (remember how eating the pulp and skin of an apple helps you digest and process the sugars from the apple's juice?). Fiber is essential for reducing your blood glucose level (Riccardi & Rivellese, 1991).

Most people who struggle with weight loss are emotional eaters. They love the taste of certain foods and find comfort in them. It's not much different than someone who drinks a lot of alcohol to drown their problems or smokes cigarettes to abate stress. People who indulge in such behaviors are trying to numb their pain.

When you have decided that you do have too much fat on your body, the first step is to make sure you're eating healthy, whole foods. Stopping yourself from eating too much of anything is the second step. That's where hormones and willpower come into play. But willpower is not reliable on its own.

If you're dealing with an extra 100 pounds or more of weight, especially if you think it's visceral fat, it may be best to consult a doctor or personal trainer. Of course, I encourage you to utilize the methods I have given you here as well. If you're facing an extra 50 pounds or less, I can easily help you.

I'm not going to insult your intelligence by telling you "all you have to do to lose weight is change your diet and exercise" because I'm sure you've heard that a thousand times before. If it were that easy, everyone would be doing it. Remember, we're looking to find the root cause, not just treat the symptoms. My mentor told me that in order to solve a problem, the first thing you have to do is ACCURATELY IDENTIFY the problem. Until you can do that, you're wasting your time.

So let's start by accurately identifying the problem. Pretend you and I are sitting across a table talking with each other, and it goes as follows:

I ask you, "What's wrong?"

You say some version of, "I'm overweight."

"What's causing you to be overweight?"

"The food I eat."

"Why do you eat the food you eat?"

"Because I'm upset, depressed, scared, lonely…" And you continue with all your "reasons."

"Why are you upset?"

Here you'll probably give me a grocery list of what's wrong.

"Why do you eat the foods you eat when you're upset?"

"Because it makes me feel better. I don't have any control over it."

"So food works for you just like alcohol works for an alcoholic, like drugs work for a drug addict, like cigarettes work for a heavy smoker, and so on. I think it's safe to say you're an emotional eater. Some people say, 'Just use willpower.' To which I reply, 'Oh yeah? The next time you have diarrhea, just use willpower to not need the bathroom.'"

In summation, you believe the problem is you're upset, depressed, lonely, scared, or some other emotion or combination of emotions.

When you eat your comfort foods, it's a "quick fix" that makes you feel better for a while. But once the "high" of the food wears off, you have to eat more to feel "better" again. The foods you choose to stress eat often have no nutritional value. You don't know what to do about the negative feedback loop you find yourself in.

If you can realize, understand, and accept that overeating is a **symptom**, not the cause of your problem, then you're on the right track to resolving it in a positive, healthy, and constructive way. What's causing you to be upset, depressed, etc.? Now, once you ask yourself this, we're getting to the root cause of the problem.

The root problem is you don't know how to deal with the negative emotions that you feel in a positive, healthy, constructive, stress-free way. If you knew how to do that, you wouldn't need the food (or alcohol, drugs, etc.) because when you faced difficult feelings and emotions, you'd use the proper tools to deal with them in a positive, healthy, constructive, stress-free way. So let's start working on that.

One extremely effective stress-managing method is called the emotional freedom technique (EFT), which is based on tapping certain acupressure points on your body to elicit a calming emotional response. In addition to helping you manage your stress, EFT can also help you lose weight. This technique helps to reprogram your subconscious beliefs in a positive, healthy, constructive, stress-free way. Healing the internal pain you feel (with this technique, mindfulness, and other coping skills) will set you on the path to your desired outcome.

The biggest mind hack I know of has to do with reprogramming your subconscious mind, effectively directing it to get on board with your desired outcome. You always want to speak positively to yourself, especially when programming your subconscious. We wouldn't want to program negative thoughts into ourselves, would we?

When you look in the mirror every day and tell yourself that you're too fat, too ugly, your nose isn't the right shape, your hands are too wide, or whatever other superficial problem you want to pick on yourself about, you are telling your subconscious mind that that's the way you want to think about yourself.

Every morning when you first get up out of bed to pee, take a few seconds and look yourself in the eyes in the mirror and say, "I am beautiful" (or "I am handsome," whichever you prefer). "I am attractive—physically, mentally, emotionally, spiritually, and sexually. I am worthy of love."

I also want you to get a small piece of paper and write out the following: "I weigh [target weight #]. I am in perfect health, and I got here in a positive, healthy, constructive, stress-free way. I love making healthy food choices and do so every day!"

Take this piece of paper and Scotch tape it to the wall next to your computer or your bed, someplace you spend a lot of time. You can even keep a copy in your purse or gym bag to look at any time you go exercise. Over time, the more you read it, the more it will sink into your subconscious. Before you know it, you'll be seeing movement toward your desired outcome and the accompanying positive effects.

This method (what I call a "target card") helped me lose 15 pounds over the last two years. My weight loss was slow, but I noticed myself gradually beginning to favor healthier food choices over time until finally the sugary sweets I'd been indulging in no longer held any appeal. Even if you're happy with your weight, you can still use this method. Just put your current weight in the blank space and hang it up. Over time, it can help change your inner (conscious and subconscious) thoughts about food, leading you to make healthier choices on a regular basis.

If you would like extra guidance, I can also recommend my End Your Emotional Eating and Sugar Addiction System. It's a detailed explanation and method for helping you identify and solve the root cause of your problem. (As a "thank you" for investing in this book, you can get the full course at a 50% discount by using code TLAHEATING50.)

Don't forget to stretch! If you have tight or stiff joints, yoga or Pilates may be an ideal method for you to reduce fat and build muscle. I aim to stretch every day. It has helped me get through winter while I've been sitting in front of the computer writing this book. Lately, I've been looking into somatic yoga and Qigong as ways to help stretch my fascia and exercise my muscles in a more gentle way. I have included my current workout/stretching routine so you can follow along with me if you want to (linked in the Additional Resources section at the end of the book).

If you're just starting out, try walking to the end of the block and slowly build to lengthening your route as you build up endurance. The whole point is to start small and build from there. I think you'll find you love it once you've done it a few times. Or, if you're more adventurous and your health permits, perhaps you can get in a hike a couple of days each week.

In warmer weather, I take a hike at least once a week and a walk almost every day. In the winter months when I can't get out much, I do short stints of walking on my walking pad, exercising with my kettlebell, and jumping on my rebounder. The bonus of using my rebounder is that it helps move lymph through my system while exercising my muscles, plus my son absolutely loves bouncing on it as well.

All three of these—my walking pad, kettlebell, and rebounder—cost me less than $250 total, and I use them so often that they are easily worth what I paid for them. (I have included links for all of them in the recommended products section at the back of the book.) If you can't afford equipment right now, walk outdoors whenever you can and lift gallon jugs filled with water until your finances allow you to buy yourself a few pieces of equipment.

Gaining Weight

If you find yourself in the opposite position, needing to GAIN weight, first, I want to ask if you have been told so by a doctor. You can't always put stock in what your loved ones say, especially in regard to your weight. For example, if it's only your Grandma who's saying, "My baby boy is too thin," to shove more spaghetti on your plate, I would take that opinion with a healthy grain of salt.

There are indeed some cases when a person may need to gain weight. However, DO NOT fall into the trap of eating empty calories and processed junk food to gain weight. All that will do is make you gain extra fat around your middle and mess with your cholesterol. Supplementing creatine monohydrate is a good way to help your body process and absorb protein, which will allow you to gain the right kind of weight and grow your muscle mass at the same time.

If you can add just 300-500 calories to your daily diet, you should be on track to steadily reaching a healthy weight for you. Try to incorporate foods such as meats that are high in protein. Such meats include ground lamb, pork chops, or steak tips (not highly processed meats such as hot dogs, pepperoni, salami, etc.). You can also increase your intake of healthy fats such as avocados, nuts, seeds, and dairy products (if you can tolerate them).

Whether you're trying to gain weight, lose weight, or maintain a weight you're happy at, you can always learn something new about managing your weight with natural methods. The information found in this chapter is also good to have on hand when your friend texts you, asking for your favorite ways to lose a few pounds before beach season. By following the advice we've gone over here, you should expect to see gradual and healthy change over time, without needing to go to extremes. Practicing being happy with the way you look (so long as it's at a weight that is healthy for your body) is the best way to cultivate lasting self-love and acceptance regarding your body image and weight.

Chapter 37: Fatigue, Brain Fog, and Adaptogens

Temporary fatigue is what happens when you stay up too late and have to get up early the next day or when some event wakes you up in the night and causes you to lose a few hours of sleep. It can also be when you took a ten-mile-long hike when you're only accustomed to hiking three miles and you feel like passing out afterward. These instances of fatigue are normal responses to overworking your body and do not require any special treatment other than adequate rest and sleep.

If you have already fallen into the trap of drinking coffee to get through the day, fear not! You can beat that need. I generally suggest people cut their coffee consumption to less than 12 ounces in the morning and drink tea for the rest of the day if they still want something caffeinated. Once you're getting proper nutrition and adequate sleep, your body won't NEED coffee to keep you awake and boost your energy levels. (However, if improved diet and sleep don't help, you may have a deeper problem that requires some diagnostic testing done by your doctor.)

Although caffeinated beverages should not be your only means for getting through the day, I don't discount a cup or two of black tea every now and then. Why? Because black tea contains L-theanine, a compound known to promote relaxation. Some people, myself included, actually benefit greatly from an afternoon cup of tea, as it can help your body process the stress you may have experienced during your morning. Simply sitting down for ten minutes to relax, slow down, and enjoy a cup of hot tea is a rejuvenating experience on a long, stressful workday.

If you are experiencing temporary fatigue or low energy (I mean the kind that lasts a week or so), even without the presentation of any other symptoms, it's possible your body is fighting off a virus. In which case, forcing yourself to get up and go for an hour-long walk at your nearest nature trail, even if you're still in your pajama pants, is going to do you more good than lying on the couch all day.

Brain fog is something almost everyone has experienced at least once, normally during or just after a bout of sickness. Have you ever been coughing, sneezing, tired, and unable to think straight while you stare at the same passage in a book that you've read over and over again? That's brain fog. If it takes you a long time to wake up in the morning or if you can't get started without a cup of coffee (or several cups), that is also brain fog rearing its ugly head. If you feel like you're drunk all the time, or most of the time, and you haven't been drinking, you're experiencing brain fog.

Brain fog is not a concern when you get it along with a host of other viral symptoms because you know that eventually the symptoms will end and you'll go back to normal. Brain fog only becomes a problem when it's chronic. Such instances may include when you repeatedly try and fail to recall a memory, when you cannot focus on a subject you've been studying, or when you unsuccessfully attempt to complete paperwork you need to get finished—when your mind simply cannot focus no matter what you do or how hard you try.

Brain fog is directly affected by your gut microbiome. Similar to when you experience fatigue, your body is either lacking a vital nutrient or the right strains of probiotics. Thus, it is unable to maintain homeostasis. What little amount of the correct nutrients you are getting is used to maintain more vital systems, like heart or liver function. Your mind doesn't technically need to be clear to do its most basic tasks, so it is not prioritized in nutrient distribution.

I'm guessing you want to have a clear brain again; I know I did during the time I was experiencing brain fog. Unsurprisingly, the first and most important step is re-establishing gut homeostasis. Following the whole foods diet outlined in this book as well as implementing the suggestions I give you in my Gut Healing Protocol will lay the foundation you need to regain your mental clarity.

Your gut is directly connected to your brain and is often called your second brain. Your **enteric nervous system**, the part of your autonomic nervous system that resides in your gut, is comprised of two thin layers of 100 million nerve cells that line your digestive tract and send signals to your actual brain (Purves, 2001). It can function independently of your brain to control the various processes of digestion. The inner lining of your small intestine can tell you that it's craving a certain food the same way your mind can. It's pretty cool to have two brains inside you, isn't it?

The two brains—your gut and your brain—talk to each other regularly and influence the operations of each other. When your gut is in good health, it is able to send important information to your brain. Likewise, your brain being in good health means it can accurately assess and act on information in a timely manner. Have you ever felt nervous and gotten a "gut feeling" about a person or situation? That's your enteric nervous system sending signals to your brain to protect you. It's been coined your "intuition," which I urge you to trust always! However, if your gut is in disarray and you're experiencing brain fog, you may not be getting these crucial signals—ones that are meant to help guide you regarding your decision-making, your health, your judgment, your path, and your safety.

If you are experiencing fatigue, brain fog, or low energy on a long-term basis, that's when you should consider seeking medical help. Go to your doctor and have a hormone level blood test done. From here, I would suggest you learn how to gauge the results for yourself. A doctor telling you that your blood test is "normal" without giving you an explanation or understanding of why it was concluded to be "normal" does you no good. If you want your body to thrive, you need to advocate for yourself and take the reins to start learning what your body actually needs.

Iron, magnesium, potassium, and zinc deficiencies are the most common culprits of fatigue. You may not be getting enough B vitamins from your diet, in which case a B-complex supplement should help you tremendously. Remember, your body requires vitamin C and copper to absorb iron from your diet, and it needs enough calcium to absorb magnesium and vice versa. Eating liver and onions once a week as part of your whole foods diet covers a lot of these bases.

Adaptogens

There are many herbalists who will hear you say that you have regular fatigue symptoms and will tell you, "What you need is an adaptogenic herb!"

An adaptogen is an herb, root, or mushroom that can be taken regularly and safely to help your body manage and adapt to stress. Adaptogens were discovered in the Western herbal paradigm during World War II, when the Russians were trying to find ways they could get their soldiers to last longer on the battlefield without giving them dangerous amphetamines (Panossian & Wikman, 2010). Several Asian herbs were tested on animals and then humans to determine whether they could make their energy last longer.

In many such studies, a control set of mice are thrown into swimming tanks, and the scientists time how long they swim around until they give up and begin drowning. They then give a second set of mice a measured amount of an adaptogenic herb and run the same test. Over time, they have figured out that certain herbs allow the mice to swim for a longer time before giving up (Kannur et al., 2008). (I don't like these methods of testing, but it's how such research has been conducted.)

After being tested on mice, these adaptogenic herbs were then tested on soldiers. Over time, certain herbs were found to be more stimulating than others, with some having more tonic-like effects. Through these studies, adaptogenic herbs, such as Eleuthero (also known as Siberian ginseng), were found to not produce more energy but to actually reduce the person's ability to feel tired (demonstrating a similar effect to caffeine in coffee). In modern times, Eleuthero has become popular with gym rats due to its ability to seemingly extend endurance during exercise.

When in a stressful situation, your body does not understand the difference between real danger and perceived danger. Your body cannot differentiate between the stress of being on the battlefield versus the stress of being on a stage. Neither can it distinguish between the stress your body experiences when running away from a mountain lion that's about to eat you versus the stress of being screamed at by your boss in a tense work environment. It's all stress—fight or flight—and your mind forces your body to deal with it in one way or another.

Your **adrenal glands** play an important role in your body's stress response, primarily through the release of adrenaline and cortisol (Johns Hopkins Medicine, 2025a). They are tiny organs that sit atop your kidneys and produce hormones that help regulate your blood pressure, metabolism, immune system, stress response, and other essential functions. Imagine them as little moist sponges that keep getting their water squeezed out every time you experience a stressful situation. What most adaptogens do is take that barely damp sponge and squeeze the hell out of it to release the last remaining drops of energy you have.

The majority of adaptogenic herbs, when taken for long periods of time, can promote burnout. The few that act as a tonic to the system, like Tulsi or Reishi mushrooms, can be safely taken for a year or more. But most adaptogens should not be taken for more than six months at most. They are a short-term remedy to be relied on for support while you are repairing the nutritional deficiencies that got you into this stress deficit in the first place. Unfortunately, many people are told adaptogens "give you energy," so they end up taking them as supplements for years upon years. After ten years of taking Eleuthero, imagine how little of your own energy bank is left inside your body. You're like a dried-up battery depending on herbs to get by.

For this reason I don't usually recommend adaptogens. I have taken Rhodiola for short periods of time, and it did help me get through those short periods of time. For example, a student trying to get through midterms or a businessman trying to complete a particularly difficult contract negotiation may turn to adaptogens to complete said task. Some herbs are great at helping you deal with this kind of stress for a month or so, but if taken any longer, they can pose serious risks to your health. To learn more about adaptogens, I highly recommend you learn more from David Winston; he literally wrote the book on them!

Fatigue, brain fog, and being plain tired suck; we've all been there before. What's important is that you identify the root cause of these issues in your life in order to effectively solve them, rather than reaching for an herbal stimulant the minute you start feeling fatigued or foggy. When you ask yourself, "Why am I feeling this way?" instead of "What can I take to stop feeling this way?" you're engaging your problem-solving skills and working toward a solution, not just looking for a temporary, quick fix. This is the path to reclaiming your energy, your focus, and your brain!

Chapter 38: Stress, Anxiety, and Depression Relief

It is likely that you have experienced some degree of stress, anxiety, and/or depression at various points in your life, at varying degrees. These feelings often occur during pivotal moments in life—during changes in relationships, career, and life stage. It is also common to experience one (or a combination) of these following a death, loss, or injury. Not a single person is immune to the stresses and strains of life. However, there are ways to cope with them. Here, we will delve into what distinguishes stress, anxiety, and depression from one another and your best options for alleviating each of their symptoms.

First, what's the difference between stress and anxiety? As defined by the American Psychological Association,

> People under stress experience mental and physical symptoms, such as irritability, anger, fatigue, muscle pain, digestive troubles, and difficulty sleeping. Anxiety, on the other hand, is defined by persistent, excessive worries that don't go away even in the absence of a stressor. (2022)

Stress is a natural human response to feeling overwhelmed or threatened, often triggering physical and emotional reactions to challenging situations. Anxiety is a persistent feeling of unease, worry, or fear about what may happen in the future. While general anxiety causes a more generalized fear regarding a number of different situations and circumstances, social anxiety revolves around interpersonal relationships and social situations.

Although symptoms of stress and anxiety are often similar, the main difference between them is that stress is situational (brought on by a particular stressor, circumstance, or event), while clinical anxiety is chronic (occurring with or without an inciting stressor, circumstance, or event). In my observation, anxiety is more influenced by your gut health than stress is. However, high levels of stress can cause gut imbalances, which can then, in turn, lead to you developing anxiety. It's a vicious cycle in this body-machine!

Today, social anxiety affects many young people especially, who, because so much of their lives have been conducted in an online space, have not been conditioned to interact with other people face-to-face. Lack of social experience, of course, puts pressure on someone when faced with highly stimulating and often overwhelming social situations, like attending a party or going to an amusement park. General anxiety, on the other hand, may cause you to worry about things like the toaster potentially burning the kitchen down or the dog peeing on the carpet because you're not home from work yet.

We live in humanity's most modern era, yet this period is a mere blink in our species' vast timeline. It was only in the 1890s that electricity became commonplace in homes, a truly recent development. In fact, 99% of human evolution and development occurred long before we even started living in villages (Ancient Origins 2019). If you consider the "modern era" to have begun roughly 250 years ago, just before industrialization, and human development to have begun about 300,000 years ago, then our "modern" existence accounts for only 0.083% of human history (Kennedy 2019). Despite this immense difference in time and technological advancement, our bodies still react to stress in fundamentally the same way. Whether you're tasked with submitting multiple copies of a report to your boss before noon or you're fleeing a lion on the Savannah, your body simulates the very same stress response.

The four primary stress (or trauma) responses your body uses to cope with perceived threats are "fight" (when you fight off your attacker), "flight" (when you run away), "freeze" (when you freeze in place and can't make your body move due to fear), and "fawn" (when you cower down to the perceived threat and do anything you can to appease it).

I don't recommend you punch your supervisor in the nose the next time he asks you to submit a report you're late on completing, nor is it a good idea to kiss his ass in every way the moment he looks at you to avoid getting yelled at. Experiencing high levels of stress can cause you to have any of these reactions, whether you consciously want to or not. Because we all experience stress and the reactions that accompany it, it's critical for the health of your entire body and your daily life that you find ways to manage your stress levels in healthy ways.

When you don't address or try to relieve your chronic stress, after enough time you can begin to experience **adrenal fatigue**. This is when your adrenal glands, which are the organs that give you your "get up and go" energy, become so tapped out that they can no longer push you any harder or provide you with energy. It's like squeezing a damp sponge; once the moisture is completely wrung out, there's nothing more you can do until you wet the sponge again. Trust me, some days I need to hear this just as much as you do: You have to relax, or you risk collapse. I'd rather let some of my to-do list fall behind for a time than end up collapsed in bed, unable to move for days because I pushed myself too hard.

Too much stress can cause hair loss, hormone imbalances, sleeplessness, stomach ulcers, and many other health problems. According to Paul Bergner (one of my favorite herbal teachers), "Stress inhibits the secretions of stomach acid and other enzymes that are necessary to digest foods and release their mineral content" (1997, p. 271). This means if you're dealing with too much stress in your life and not doing anything to mitigate it, your body may not be able to absorb the nutrition from your food.

Surprisingly, 90% of the serotonin—a key neurotransmitter responsible for feelings of happiness and well-being—is manufactured in your gut, not your brain (Bektaş et al., 2020). If your gut is in dysbiosis (in which there are considerably more bad microbes than good ones), it is going to affect your mood significantly and can be a major precursor to depression. My friend Cheryl Major and I combined her experience treating chronic depression and my knowledge of herbalism to craft a class to help you heal your depression symptoms naturally with food and herbs. You can access our class, Fight Depression With Food, by following the link in the Additional Resources section at the end of the book.

Depression is a mood disorder that causes a persistent feeling of sadness, loss of interest in activities, and behavioral changes that can affect whether or not a person wants to participate in society or their own life. Depression can manifest in several levels of severity. There are natural things you can do to improve or relieve depression, depending on what level you're experiencing. Serious depression that results in thoughts of self-harm or suicide should be addressed by a psychiatrist immediately. It will be up to you to discern whether any of the dietary changes, herbs, or supplements I talk about here are worth incorporating into your life based on your own desires and the potential interaction with any medication you are currently taking.

When you are struggling with stress, anxiety, or depression, it becomes all the more daunting to regain control of your health. It may seem hopeless, especially when you do not experience immediate results from improving your diet (or supplementation). If you can stick with your new nutrition goals and employ the stress-reduction techniques we cover in this chapter, with time and consistency, you will begin to feel better. It took a long time for you to get to the place where you are right now (physically, mentally, and emotionally), so it can take a while to see positive, substantial, and lasting improvement. Trust and know that your problem is fixable—there is a light at the end of the tunnel.

When my Facebook page got hacked, my stress levels went through the roof. I depended on that page for my business and income. I can't begin to imagine how much more stress I would have been under if I were dealing with anxious feelings, panic attacks, or depression on top of what I was already feeling while dealing with keeping my business afloat.

I've had two panic attacks in my life (that I can recall). They both occurred before I healed my mental health, so they were experienced by the old me, with my old mental programming and hang-ups. That woman died three years ago. The new me, thankfully, doesn't have anxiety. Sure, I occasionally worry about things, but it's never enough to stop me from living my life—continuing to strive toward what I want in my future. The new me, who is running my own business, even with my renewed mood and emotional health, is stressed as hell at times!

Having told you a little about my mental health journey, I'd like to give you some options to help you manage your stress, anxiety, and depression. I can only tell you how the following herbs, supplements, and techniques have worked for me along with the effects they are generally expected to have. I can't promise any of these solutions will be right for you, but I can assure you that they are a much safer first option to try compared to pharmaceutical medications.

To preface the solutions, we must discuss what your options are if you are currently taking a medication to treat your mental health. I have been asked by several clients how they can wean themselves off their anxiety or depression medications. Please discuss this with your doctor first to let them know you're interested in reducing or eliminating your meds because it needs to be done gradually. However, from a mental standpoint, the first step to being able to stop your medication is to accurately identify what's causing your stress, anxiety, or depression.

Until you find a way to deal with the cause in a positive, healthy, constructive, stress-free way, then all you're doing is finding a magic pill that will deaden the pain so you can continue the lifestyle that led you to the point you're at now. If you choose to take the magic pill rather than find a solution that addresses the root cause of the stress, your symptoms will continue to worsen. The continued stress could inevitably lead to a heart attack or cancer (both of which can be fatal). Chronic stress forces you to contend with the life you're living and the choices you're making, even if the result of your choices is illness or death.

Weaning off a medication depends on a lot of factors: how long you've been taking the meds, how much you are taking, the type of meds, your lifestyle, and your dedication to resolving the issues that led to you being on medication. Some medications are stronger than others, which is why it's important to know more about the process from your doctor.

There are herbs and supplements that can help ease your stress, anxiety, and/or depression, but in most cases they aren't going to affect your body and mood as drastically as a pharmaceutical does. That's why it's critical that you slowly wean off your medication while implementing other methods that can help you manage your mental health. If you have SEVERE anxiety or depression, I suggest you speak with a physician. Herbs may not be your best choice for a number of reasons.

Please know that the following herbal suggestions are offered from a clinical perspective rather than from a personal one. I have not suffered with chronic anxiety or depression. While I have worked with these herbs for various purposes (including supporting my mental health), I have not personally used them to treat clinical anxiety or depression. That being said, these are the herbs I would recommend to someone who is looking to do so.

When treating anxiety or depression, you want to research **nervine herbs**, which affect your nervous system. They come in various strengths, with varying affinities for treating anxiety, depression, nervousness, restlessness, sleeplessness, and stress. Remember, each herb has many different medicinal constituents inside it that can affect more than just your nervous system, so please do more in-depth research on any herb before you start taking it medicinally.

Nervine herbs to support mental health and general well-being:

Chamomile *(Matricaria recutita)*: an herb most commonly known for helping you fall asleep at night. It can be taken during the day for its relaxing properties as well. Additionally, it can be an ally in healing your stomach and reducing inflammation in your body. You don't have to grow it yourself or spend tons of money on big bags of it. It's easy to get a box of chamomile tea at just about ANY store. The longer you steep the chamomile, the better, since its medicinal properties are drawn out and increased with longer exposure to the water. You can even use two tea bags if you like. Chamomile can also be taken in tincture form. It is quite easy to grow if you have some garden space, and it tastes wonderful fresh.

Holy basil *(Ocimum sanctum)*: my favorite herb when it comes to relaxing tension, stress, and anxiety—also known by the name "tulsi." It protects the heart from stress, lowers blood pressure and cholesterol levels, and can help stabilize blood sugar levels. This herb increases joy and happiness and induces a feeling that all will be alright.

Lavender *(Lavandula officinalis)*: a relaxing nervine for tension and anxiety. It helps in lifting your mood and can be mildly antidepressant—especially helpful for high-strung, nervous people. It can also help you or a child fall asleep. You can add it in your tea blend, but be sure to not add too much because it can cause your tea to taste off-putting. Many people swear by rubbing a dab of lavender oil on the bottoms of their feet to aid sleep. This definitely helped my kids fall asleep when they were little.

Lemon balm *(Melissa officinalis)*: helpful for general anxiety, nervousness that affects the heart, sadness, and depression. It is also calming and helps aid sleep. I add this to thyroid and uterus support blends. It smells like lemon, tastes mildly lemony, and grows with insane abundance on my farm.

Motherwort *(Leonurus cardiaca)*: a very strong nervine that can help you if you have anxiety or stress related to your relationship with your mother (yes, I'm serious). This herb drops your blood pressure quickly! It's not meant to be taken in place of blood pressure medication, but it can potentially be incorporated into a natural treatment plan for normalizing blood pressure. However, use caution before you start adding motherwort to your regime, especially if you're dealing with blood pressure issues.

For reference, I naturally have low blood pressure. The first time I took this, I didn't realize how drastic the effect would be. Taking a half dropperful of this tincture made me feel like I was sinking into a big fluffy feather bed that I did not want to get up from.

Passionflower *(Passiflora incarnata)*: a relaxing nervine that can help quiet the mind if you have racing thoughts preventing you from falling asleep. It is a VERY safe choice of herb for adults and children alike. I add this to my sleepy teas and tinctures. It generally has a pleasant taste.

Skullcap *(Scutellaria lateriflora)*: a relaxing nervine that can ease chronic insomnia or stress. If you have an inability to pay attention or are overly sensitive to external stimuli, such as light and sound, taking skullcap may benefit you greatly. To me, taking a dose of skullcap tincture feels like you're a lit candle that is being snuffed out. I LOVE this herb! You can get some from Mountain Rose Herbs if you want to try it for yourself.

Now that we have covered the herbs that can help manage your mental health, let's talk supplementation. DHEA (dehydroepiandrosterone) is a hormone produced by the adrenal glands that helps modulate your body's stress response. You produce some on your own, but if you are regularly dealing with high cortisol levels, it may be helpful for you to supplement. I have been taking DHEA as a supplement for several years now, as a naturopathic doctor suggested it could help me manage my overall stress levels.

I had a blood test done a few months ago. Upon seeing the results, my doctor said that my DHEA levels were much higher than she expected them to be. She was concerned I may have a tumor on my adrenal glands with levels this high. I told her I had been supplementing with 100 mg of DHEA daily. She asked me to stop taking it for a month and then have my blood retested.

During the month I was not taking DHEA, I experienced sadness, fear, anxiety, and depression—all things I rarely experienced before. I did not know what was wrong with me, but I attributed it to low vitamin D (since it was winter). Eventually, I went and got my blood retested, and to my surprise (and the doctor's), my natural DHEA levels were dangerously low. She said, "No wonder you were on the supplement! Why don't you cut it in half, though, to be safe?"

Now, instead of taking a 100 mg capsule in the morning, I take a 25 mg tablet in the morning and a 25 mg tablet in the afternoon. I tried taking 50 mg in the morning, but I would feel anxious by the evening, so I swapped it out for half and half and am doing great now.

If you want to try this method, I suggest you start with 25 mg a day to see how it makes you feel. Alternatively, you could get a blood panel done and ask for your DHEA levels to be tested. For reference, anything under 100 is quite low.

In addition to taking DHEA, I started taking a stress relief supplement a few months ago, which is made with saffron (a powerful stress support herb). It has greatly helped reduce my overall stress levels. If you want to give it a try, it's Silver Fern™ Brand's Stress Complex.

Other methods I utilize for stress relief:

I frequently utilize EFT (the emotional freedom technique) to deal with feelings of worry or stress. EFT focuses on tapping acupressure points on the body in a repetitive fashion while repeating your problem, followed by a solution. In effect, the tapping and verbal looping release emotional stress and induce a sense of well-being, clarity, and calm in your mental state. Nick Ortner, Brad Yates, and many other practitioners are available to guide you through EFT on YouTube for free.

Three of the best ways to naturally reduce stress are absolutely free: standing or walking barefoot on the ground (preferably on grass or some other cushy groundcover), hugging a tree, and cuddling with a loved one or pet. These three activities increase dopamine and oxytocin levels in your body (Spiller, 2024) and are better than any drug you could take.

Exercise, something as simple as taking a walk down a nature trail where you can hear birds singing and see some greenery, releases mood-boosting endorphins and increases circulation in your body. Regularly exercising can help you get better quality sleep at night, which in turn will allow your brain to rest and reset. This is crucially important since sleep deprivation is a major contributor to worsened depression.

For all of its many benefits, get outdoors when you can. As previously discussed, sun exposure is vital to naturally producing necessary levels of vitamin D in your body, as well as helping keep your circadian rhythm in balance. Additionally, it's been scientifically proven that hearing birdsong and breathing fresh air near trees is relaxing to humans (Hrustic, 2025). Birds wouldn't be singing if they were trying to escape danger; singing is a sign that all is well in their world, so it should be for us too!

It's important to remember that stress, anxiety, and depression are all fixable and, in many cases, can be remedied without medication. However, natural solutions are only effective when you approach your current situation from a holistic perspective, slowly implementing these changes over time. Please don't stop taking your medication cold turkey in favor of taking the herbs I have suggested here! Ease yourself off slowly with the help of your doctor, as stopping cold turkey can cause serious side effects in many cases. Utilizing your personal arsenal of natural solutions will have you feeling better before you know it. There's no need to rush your health.

Conclusion

I know you have the power to heal yourself—physically, mentally, emotionally, spiritually, and sexually. I did it, and you can too!

I wrote this book so I could help people heal THEMSELVES.

Your current lifestyle, the way you've been living for the last 10, 20, 30, or more years, has determined what your health looks like right now. But where you are right now does not have to be permanent. The people who do the best with any kind of advice are those who are interested in continual self-improvement. When you realize, understand, and accept that the only way to cure yourself long-term is to adopt a completely different lifestyle, you put yourself back in control of your life.

To suffice, lifestyle is broken down into the following areas:

- What you eat (and the state of your microbiome)
- Your exercise habits
- Your faith and beliefs
- Your self-image

The total improvement of your physical health is not just a matter of a few diet changes. You must incorporate mental health into your healing to address mental and emotional blocks that are very likely affecting your overall health. The last thing I want you to do is switch your poor eating habits to an alcohol or drug problem in an attempt to cope. Unless you find a way to face your emotions, past, and mental programming, you'll just end up trading one addiction or problem for another, with your deeper issues never being resolved.

When you get upset, more often than not, your stomach also becomes upset. When you intuitively feel something is wrong about a person or situation, you get a "gut feeling." When you feel nervous, your hands may shake, your face may flush, and you may sweat more than usual. Your emotions have a much greater influence over your physical body than you sometimes give them credit for. Think of the saying "mind over matter." It tracks because what you do with your mind matters.

If you combine mental and emotional therapies (EFT, meditation, remote healing, somatic therapy, subconscious reprogramming, etc.) with a well-rounded, complete, whole foods-based diet, you will have laid the groundwork to heal yourself from the inside out. Healing yourself physically, mentally, emotionally, spiritually, sexually, financially, creatively, and artistically—now that is what I call a complete lifestyle change.

YOU have the power in your hands, mind, and heart. You also have ample resources to help you along the journey.

Yes, sometimes you should consult a doctor. You're never going to cheat death. When the universe decides it's your time to go, it's your time to go. But you DO have control over how you care for yourself in this moment. Make health-conscious choices that will give you the best quality of life and that don't shorten your life expectancy.

It took me over twenty years to learn everything that we have covered in this book, mostly through experience but also through plenty of studying. It is my hope that in reading this, you now have a head start to taking control of your health or a starting place to resolving any health issue you are currently facing. I strived to impart authentic, learned wisdom that you could apply to your life or give to your kid before they step out into the world on their own and are forced to learn all this stuff the hard way.

I did not want to approach this project as if I were writing a report for English class. I have a BA in English; I remember writing hundreds of papers like that. For this reason, I provided you with the resources I used to learn the basics so that you can dive deeper into each subject if you wish to do so. I also included citations to useful research so that you can gain an understanding of how certain scientific conclusions were reached.

The end of this book has a list of books and resources that I trust. It has taken me many years to figure out who to trust and the best places to look for reliable health information. I'm always learning, so it is my intention to update this list in the future. Additionally, I have included pages with all other resources and products mentioned throughout the text so you can easily look them up for yourself. (Some of the products I recommend in this book can be purchased through my affiliate link. If you order something through one of my links, I will receive a small commission at no extra cost to you.)

I expect you found at least one thing you can take away from this book, whether that be something you learned that you didn't know before or something you had learned long ago and forgotten that I reminded you of. My aim was to convey the information I know to you in the only way I know how: directly, truthfully, and in easy-to-comprehend language. You don't have to be a professional herbalist, nutritionist, or doctor to become knowledgeable about your health.

You will learn best from a teacher that "calls to" or "speaks to" you. Your vibe matches your tribe! You will be drawn to those who present their information and knowledge in a way that you are able to absorb and comprehend. For example, while I greatly respect and admire Rosemary Gladstar and Matthew Wood, both of whom are knowledgeable herbalists, my brain has not enjoyed their particular teaching styles as much as some of the other herbalists out there. Every herb teacher has their own style; you want to learn from the teacher (and style) that suits you because that means you will retain the information better.

If you're wondering where I started my herbalism education, I attended the Heart of Herbs Herbal School. I have also studied with and would recommend the School of Evolutionary Herbalism as well as the Acorn School of Herbal Medicine. I also listen to several podcasts Including HerbRally, Herbs with Rosalee, and the Commonwealth Holistic Herbalism Podcast.

I will be publishing another book soon that covers my incredible journey toward getting my mental health for the first time in my life, and how you can get it too. Follow me on social media for updates!

If you're interested in my particular teaching style or services or would like me to teach or speak at your event, don't hesitate to reach out. And if you enjoyed my book, please write a review! I genuinely appreciate it.

References

1. Abdi, F., Ozgoli, G., & Rahnemaie, F. S. (2019). A systematic review of the role of vitamin D and calcium in premenstrual syndrome. *Obstetrics & Gynecology Science*, *62*(2), 73–86. https://doi.org/10.5468/ogs.2019.62.2.73

2. Al-Atif, H. (2022). Collagen Supplements for Aging and Wrinkles: a Paradigm Shift in the Field of Dermatology and Cosmetics. *Dermatology Practical & Conceptual*, *12*(1), e2022018. https://doi.org/10.5826/dpc.1201a18

3. Alvergne, A., & Lummaa, V. (2010). Does the contraceptive pill alter mate choice in humans? *Trends in Ecology & Evolution*, *25*(3), 171–179. https://doi.org/10.1016/j.tree.2009.08.003

4. American Kidney Fund. (2024, February 12). *Herbal supplements and chronic kidney disease (CKD).* American Kidney Fund. https://www.kidneyfund.org/treatments/medicines-kidney-disease/herbal-supplements-and-chronic-kidney-disease-ckd

5. American Psychological Association. (2022, February 14). *What's The Difference Between Stress and Anxiety?* Apa.org; American Psychological Association. https://www.apa.org/topics/stress/anxiety-difference

6. Ancient Origins. (c. 2019). *The Stone Age: The First 99 Percent of Human History*. Ancient Origins. https://www.ancient-origins.net/human-origins-science/stone-age-0012559

7. Ansary, J., Forbes-Hernández, T. Y., Gil, E., Cianciosi, D., Zhang, J., Elexpuru-Zabaleta, M., Simal-Gandara, J., Giampieri, F., & Battino, M. (2020). Potential Health Benefit of Garlic Based on Human Intervention Studies: A Brief Overview. *Antioxidants*, *9*(7), 619. https://doi.org/10.3390/antiox9070619

8. Bargagli, M., Tio, M. C., Waikar, S. S., & Ferraro, P. M. (2020). Dietary Oxalate Intake and Kidney Outcomes. *Nutrients*, *12*(9), 2673. https://doi.org/10.3390/nu12092673

9. Beck, V., Rohr, U., & Jungbauer, A. (2005). Phytoestrogens derived from red clover: an alternative to estrogen replacement therapy? *The Journal of Steroid Biochemistry and Molecular Biology*, *94*(5), 499–518. https://doi.org/10.1016/j.jsbmb.2004.12.038

10. Bektaş , A., Erdal, H., Ulusoy, M., & Uzbay, I. T. (2020). Does Seratonin in the intestines make you happy? *The Turkish Journal of Gastroenterology*, *31*(10), 721–723. https://doi.org/10.5152/tjg.2020.19554

11. Bennett, R. R. (2013, July 2). *The Gift of Goldenrod.* Robin Rose Bennett. https://www.robinrosebennett.com/musings/resources/the-gift-of-goldenrod

12. Berg, S. (2024, January 23). *Massive study uncovers how much exercise is needed to live longer.* American Medical Association. https://www.ama-assn.org/delivering-care/prevention-wellness/massive-study-uncovers-how-much-exercise-needed-live-longer

13. Bergner, P. (1997). *The Healing Power of Minerals, Special Nutrients, and Trace Elements* (p. 271). Prima Lifestyles.

14. Bhusal, K. K., Magar, S. K., Thapa, R., Lamsal, A., Bhandari, S., Maharjan, R., Shrestha, S., & Shrestha, J. (2022). Nutritional and pharmacological importance of stinging nettle (Urtica dioica L.): A review. *Heliyon*, *8*(6), e09717. https://doi.org/10.1016/j.heliyon.2022.e09717

15. Bischoff, S. C., Barbara, G., Buurman, W., Ockhuizen, T., Schulzke, J.-D., Serino, M., Tilg, H., Watson, A., & Wells, J. M. (2014). Intestinal permeability – a new target for disease prevention and therapy. *BMC Gastroenterology*, *14*(1), 189. https://doi.org/10.1186/s12876-014-0189-7

16. Blaak, E. (2001). Gender Differences in Fat Metabolism. *Current Opinion in Clinical Nutrition and Metabolic Care*, *4*(6), 499–502. https://doi.org/10.1097/00075197-200111000-00006

17. Bowden, J., & Sinatra, S. T. (2020). *The Great Cholesterol Myth, Revised and Expanded: Why Lowering Your Cholesterol Won't Prevent Heart Disease—and the Statin-Free Plan that Will.* Fair Winds Press.

18. Brock, S. (2024, April 8). *What is Fiber and Why is it Important for the Microbiome?* Stanford Lifestyle Medicine. https://healthy.kaiserpermanente.org/health-wellness/healtharticle.ask-a-doctor-is-juicing-healthy

19. Buralli, R. J., Dultra, A. F., & Ribeiro, H. (2020). Respiratory and Allergic Effects in Children Exposed to Pesticides—A Systematic Review. *International Journal of Environmental Research and Public Health*, *17*(8), 2740. https://doi.org/10.3390/ijerph17082740

20. Burrows, P., & Griffiths, P. (2002). Do baby walkers delay onset of walking in young children? *British Journal of Community Nursing*, *7*(11), 581–586. https://doi.org/10.12968/bjcn.2002.7.11.10889

21. Çalişkan, N., Bulut, H., & Konan, A. (2016). The Effect of Warm Water Intake on Bowel Movements in the Early Postoperative Stage of Patients Having Undergone Laparoscopic Cholecystectomy: A Randomized Controlled Trial. *Gastroenterology Nursing, 39*(5), 340–347. https://doi.org/10.1097/SGA.0000000000000181

22. Carr, A. C., & Maggini, S. (2017). Vitamin C and Immune Function. *Nutrients, 9*(11), 1211. https://doi.org/10.3390/nu9111211

23. Cazzola, R., Della Porta, M., Manoni, M., Iotti, S., Pinotti, L., & Maier, J. A. (2020). Going to the roots of reduced magnesium dietary intake: A tradeoff between climate changes and sources. *Heliyon, 6*(11), e05390. https://doi.org/10.1016/j.heliyon.2020.e05390

24. Centers for Disease Control and Prevention. (2024, February 20). *About Genital Herpes.* Cdc.gov. https://www.cdc.gov/herpes/about/index.html

25. Chesak, J. (2024, February 13). *I Tried 12 Weeks of Strength Training For Perimenopause & Here's What Happened.* Mindbodygreen. https://www.mindbodygreen.com/articles/strength-training-for-perimenopause?srsltid=AfmBOopSdMDnN4zu1-2ihem40fAw3xC1IZOMlCD05WWdSf2mazYbCOq6

26. Clare, B. A., Conroy, R. S., & Spelman, K. (2009). The Diuretic Effect in Human Subjects of an Extract of Taraxacum officinale Folium over a Single Day. *Journal of Alternative and Complementary Medicine, 15*(8), 929–934. https://doi.org/10.1089/acm.2008.0152

27. Cobey, K. D., Havlíček, J., Klapilová, K., & Roberts, S. C. (2015). Hormonal Contraceptive Use During Relationship Formation and Sexual Desire During Pregnancy. *Archives of Sexual Behavior, 45*(8), 2117–2122. https://doi.org/10.1007/s10508-015-0662-6

28. Cotton Australia. (2020, May 12). *Soil Your Undies Experiment.* YouTube. https://www.youtube.com/watch?v=Jbn8ogSyZ3o

29. Davis, W. (2019). *Wheat Belly: Lose the Wheat, Lose the Weight, and Find Your Path Back to Health* (pp. 23–24). Rodale Books. (Original work published 2011)

30. Dawson-Hughes, B. (2004). Racial/ethnic considerations in making recommendations for vitamin D for adult and elderly men and women. *The American Journal of Clinical* Nutrition, 80(6), 1763S1766S. https://doi.org/10.1093/ajcn/80.6.1763s

31. Douda, D. (2017, November 7). *Mayo Clinic Minute: Is Alzheimer's Type 3 diabetes?* Https://Newsnetwork.mayoclinic.org.

https://newsnetwork.mayoclinic.org/discussion/mayo-clinic-minute-is-alzheimers-type-3-diabetes/

32. Dr. Ida Rolf Institute. (2019). *What is Rolfing?* Rolf.org. https://www.rolf.org/rolfing.php

33. Earp, B. D. (2015). Do the Benefits of Male Circumcision Outweigh the Risks? A Critique of the Proposed CDC Guidelines. *Frontiers in Pediatrics*, *3*(18). https://doi.org/10.3389/fped.2015.00018

34. EBSCO CAM Review Board. (2024). *Wild yam in therapeutics.* EBSCO Information Services. https://www.ebsco.com/research-starters/health-and-medicine/wild-yam-therapeutics

35. Ely, P. H. (2018). Is psoriasis a bowel disease? Successful treatment with bile acids and bioflavonoids suggests it is. *Clinics in Dermatology*, *36*(3), 376–389. https://doi.org/10.1016/j.clindermatol.2018.03.011

36. Fisher, J. (2024, August 13). *Lifestyle strategies to help prevent natural age-related decline in testosterone - Harvard Health.* Harvard Health. https://www.health.harvard.edu/mens-health/lifestyle-strategies-to-help-prevent-natural-age-related-decline-in-testosterone

37. Guo, E. (2021, February 20). *Vitamin Supplements: Vital or Superfluous?* The Public Health Advocate. https://pha.studentorg.berkeley.edu/2021/02/20/vitamin-supplements-vital-or-superfluous/

38. Harcourt, L. (2024, February 5). *Can magnesium impact hormone health and PMS?* Holland & Barrett. https://www.hollandandbarrett.com/the-health-hub/vitamins-and-supplements/minerals/magnesium/magnesium-benefits-hormones/

39. Hardin, B. D., Kelman, B. J., & Saxon, A. (2003). Adverse Human Health Effects Associated with Molds in the Indoor Environment. *Journal of Occupational and Environmental Medicine*, *45*(5), 470–478. https://doi.org/10.1097/00043764-200305000-00006

40. Harvard Health Publishing. (n.d.). *Testosterone: What it is and how it affects your health.* Harvard Health. https://www.health.harvard.edu/staying-healthy/testosterone--what-it-does-and-doesnt-do

41. Hill, S. E. (2019). *This Is Your Brain on Birth Control: The Surprising Science of Women, Hormones, and the Law of Unintended Consequences* (p. 7). Avery.

42. Hill, S. E. (2020, February 10). *Is Sexy in the Eye of the Pill-Taker?* Behavioral Scientist. https://behavioralscientist.org/quality-sex-relationships-birth-control-pill-research-effects/

43. Hirata, J. D., Swiersz, L. M., Zell, B., Small, R., & Ettinger, B. (1997). Does dong quai have estrogenic effects in postmenopausal women? A double-blind, placebo-controlled trial. *Fertility and Sterility*, *68*(6), 981–986. https://doi.org/10.1016/s0015-0282(97)00397-x

44. Holland, J. (2024, November 4). *New study finds associations between use of skin care products and exposure to potential developmental toxicants*. College of Public Health. https://publichealth.gmu.edu/news/2024-09/new-study-finds-associations-between-use-skin-care-products-and-exposure-potential

45. Horrocks, L. A., & Yeo, Y. K. (1999). Health benefits of docosahexaenoic acid (DHA). *Pharmacological Research*, *40*(3), 211–225. https://doi.org/10.1006/phrs.1999.0495

46. Hrustic, A. (2025, May 14). *Listening to birds sing really does soothe your brain. Here's why*. National Geographic. https://www.nationalgeographic.com/health/article/birds-sing-brain-mental-health

47. Huda, H. S., Majid, N. B. A., Chen, Y., Adnan, M., Ashraf, S. A., Roszko, M., Bryła, M., Kieliszek, M., & Sasidharan, S. (2024). Exploring the ancient roots and modern global brews of tea and herbal beverages: A comprehensive review of origins, types, health benefits, market dynamics, and future trends. *Food Science & Nutrition*, *12*(10), 6938–6955. https://doi.org/10.1002/fsn3.4346

48. Hutchison , M. (2021, October 4). *How to Make a Mushroom Double Extraction*. Mountain Rose Herbs. https://blog.mountainroseherbs.com/mushroom-double-extraction

49. Institute for Quality and Efficiency in Health Care. (2024, May 28). *In brief: How does the thyroid gland work?* National Library of Medicine. https://www.ncbi.nlm.nih.gov/books/NBK279388/

50. Jadidi, A., Rezaei Ashtiani, A., Khanmohamadi Hezaveh, A., & Aghaepour, S. M. (2022). Therapeutic effects of magnesium and vitamin B6 in alleviating the symptoms of restless legs syndrome: a randomized controlled clinical trial. *BMC Complementary Medicine and Therapies*, *23*(1). https://doi.org/10.1186/s12906-022-03814-8

51. Jahdi, F., Khabbaz, A. H., Kashian, M., Taghizadeh, M., & Haghani, H. (2018). The impact of calendula ointment on cesarean wound healing: A randomized controlled clinical trial. *Journal of Family Medicine and Primary Care*, *7*(5), 893–897. https://doi.org/10.4103/jfmpc.jfmpc_121_17

52. Jenko Pražnikar, Z., Mohorko, N., Gmajner, D., Kenig, S., & Petelin, A. (2023). Effects of Four Different Dietary Fibre Supplements on Weight Loss and

Lipid and Glucose Serum Profiles during Energy Restriction in Patients with Traits of Metabolic Syndrome: A Comparative, Randomized, Placebo-Controlled Study. *Foods*, *12*(11), 2122. https://doi.org/10.3390/foods12112122

53. Johns Hopkins Medicine. (n.d.). *Muscle Pain: It May Actually Be Your Fascia*. Hopkinsmedicine.org. Retrieved May 28, 2025, from https://www.hopkinsmedicine.org/health/wellness-and-prevention/muscle-pain-it-may-actually-be-your-fascia

54. Johns Hopkins Medicine. (2019). *Hormones and the Endocrine System*. Hopkinsmedicine.org. https://www.hopkinsmedicine.org/health/conditions-and-diseases/hormones-and-the-endocrine-system

55. Johns Hopkins Medicine. (2021). *Intermittent fasting: What is it, and how does it work?* Hopkinsmedicine.org. https://www.hopkinsmedicine.org/health/wellness-and-prevention/intermittent-fasting-what-is-it-and-how-does-it-work

56. Johns Hopkins Medicine. (2023, August 1). *Cayenne*. Hopkinsmedicine.org. https://johnshopkinshealthcare.staywellsolutionsonline.com/19,Cayenne

57. Johns Hopkins Medicine. (2025a). *Adrenal Glands*. Hopkinsmedicine.org. https://www.hopkinsmedicine.org/health/conditions-and-diseases/adrenal-glands

58. Johns Hopkins Medicine. (2025b). *Liver: Anatomy and Functions*. Hopkinsmedicine.org. https://www.hopkinsmedicine.org/health/conditions-and-diseases/liver-anatomy-and-functions

59. Kaloti, R. (2021, November 11). *10 Health Issues Caused By Bad Oral Health*. West 85th Dental. https://west85thdental.com/10-health-issues-caused-by-bad-oral-health/

60. Kaminski, P. (2016, January 14). *Hawthorn: A Special Affinity to the Heart*. Flower Essence Services. https://www.fesflowers.com/hawthorn-special-affinity-heart/

61. Kanellopoulos, A. K., & Costello, S. E. (2024). The effects of prolonged pacifier use on language development in infants and toddlers. *Frontiers in Psychology*, *15*, 1349323. https://doi.org/10.3389/fpsyg.2024.1349323

62. Kannur, D. M., Kulkarni, A. A., Paranjpe, M. P., & Navangul, M. V. (2008). Screening of Antistress Properties of Herbal Extracts and Adaptogenic Agents – A Review . *Pharmacognosy Reviews*, *2*(3), 95–101. https://www.phcogrev.com/sites/default/files/PhcogRev-2-3-95.pdf

63. Kapper, C., Oppelt, P., Ganhör, C., Gyunesh, A. A., Arbeithuber, B., Stelzl, P., & Rezk-Füreder, M. (2024). Minerals and the Menstrual Cycle: Impacts on Ovulation and Endometrial Health. *Nutrients*, *16*(7), 1008. https://doi.org/10.3390/nu16071008

64. Kennedy, L. (2019, September 27). *The Prehistoric Ages: How Humans Lived Before Written Records*. History. A&E Television Networks. Retrieved August 27, 2025, from https://www.history.com/articles/prehistoric-ages-timeline

65. Khoo, H. E., Azlan, A., Tang, S. T., & Lim, S. M. (2017). Anthocyanidins and anthocyanins: Colored Pigments as food, Pharmaceutical ingredients, and the Potential Health Benefits. *Food & Nutrition Research*, *61*(1), 1361779. https://doi.org/10.1080/16546628.2017.1361779

66. Kil, M. S., Kim, C. W., & Kim, S. S. (2013). Analysis of Serum Zinc and Copper Concentrations in Hair Loss. *Annals of Dermatology*, *25*(4), 405–409. https://doi.org/10.5021/ad.2013.25.4.405

67. Kim, T. W., Jeong, J.-H., & Hong, S.-C. (2015). The Impact of Sleep and Circadian Disturbance on Hormones and Metabolism. *International Journal of Endocrinology*, *2015*(591729), 1–9. https://doi.org/10.1155/2015/591729

68. Kincaid, C., Jones, D. J., Sterrett, E., & McKee, L. (2012). A review of parenting and adolescent sexual behavior: The moderating role of gender. *Clinical Psychology Review*, *32*(3), 177–188. https://doi.org/10.1016/j.cpr.2012.01.002

69. Kolanu, B. R., Vadakedath, S., Boddula, V., & Kandi, V. (2020). Activities of Serum Magnesium and Thyroid Hormones in Pre-, Peri-, and Post-menopausal Women. *Cureus*, *12*(1), e6554. https://doi.org/10.7759/cureus.6554

70. Komesaroff, P. A., Black, C. V., Cable, V., & Sudhir, K. (2001). Effects of wild yam extract on menopausal symptoms, lipids and sex hormones in healthy menopausal women. *Climacteric: The Journal of the International Menopause Society*, *4*(2), 144–150. https://pubmed.ncbi.nlm.nih.gov/11428178/

71. LaMotte, S. (2025, February 3). *Human brain samples contain an entire spoon's worth of nanoplastics, study says.* CNN. https://www.cnn.com/2025/02/03/health/plastics-inside-human-brain-wellness/index.html

72. Lee, S. Y., Lee, E., Park, Y. M., & Hong, S. J. (2018). Microbiome in the Gut-Skin Axis in Atopic Dermatitis. *Allergy, Asthma & Immunology Research*, *10*(4), 354–362. https://doi.org/10.4168/aair.2018.10.4.354

73. Ma, X., Nan, F., Liang, H., Shu, P., Fan, X., Song, X., Hou, Y., & Zhang, D. (2022). Excessive intake of sugar: An accomplice of inflammation. *Frontiers in Immunology*, *13*, 988481. https://doi.org/10.3389/fimmu.2022.988481

74. Matar, A., Abdelnaem, N., & Camilleri, M. (2025). Bone Broth Benefits: How Its Nutrients Fortify Gut Barrier in Health and Disease. *Digestive Diseases and Sciences*, *70*(6), 1951–1961. https://doi.org/10.1007/s10620-025-08997-x

75. Mayo Clinic Staff. (2023, August 26). *Exercise: 7 Benefits of Regular Physical Activity*. Mayo Clinic; Mayo Foundation for Medical Education and Research. https://www.mayoclinic.org/healthy-lifestyle/fitness/in-depth/exercise/art-20048389

76. Mayo Clinic Staff. (2024, March 14). *Oral health: A window to your overall health*. Mayo Clinic. https://www.mayoclinic.org/healthy-lifestyle/adult-health/in-depth/dental/art-20047475

77. McMains, V. (2024, May 8). *Healthy Mouth, Healthy Body*. National Institute of Dental and Craniofacial Research. https://www.nidcr.nih.gov/news-events/nidcr-news/2024/healthy-mouth-healthy-body

78. Morrison, R. M., Buzby, J. C., & Wells, H. F. (2010, March 1). *Guess Who's Turning 100? Tracking a Century of American Eating | Economic Research Service*. Usda.gov. https://www.ers.usda.gov/amber-waves/2010/march/guess-who-s-turning-100-tracking-a-century-of-american-eating

79. Mueller, N. T., Bakacs, E., Combellick, J., Grigoryan, Z., & Dominguez-Bello, M. G. (2015). The infant microbiome development: mom matters. *Trends in Molecular Medicine*, *21*(2), 109–117. https://doi.org/10.1016/j.molmed.2014.12.002

80. National Institute of Arthritis and Musculoskeletal and Skin Diseases. (2023, May). *Calcium and Vitamin D: Important for Bone Health*. National Institute of Arthritis and Musculoskeletal and Skin Diseases. https://www.niams.nih.gov/health-topics/calcium-and-vitamin-d-important-bone-health

81. National Institute of Diabetes and Digestive and Kidney Diseases. (2017, December). *Your Digestive System & How It Works*. National Institute of Diabetes and Digestive and Kidney Diseases. https://www.niddk.nih.gov/health-information/digestive-diseases/digestive-system-how-it-works

82. National Institute of Diabetes and Digestive and Kidney Diseases. (2018, June). *Your Kidneys & How They Work*. National Institute of Diabetes and Digestive and Kidney Diseases. https://www.niddk.nih.gov/health-information/kidney-disease/kidneys-how-they-work

83. National Institute of Environmental Health Sciences. (2024, July 22). *Endocrine Disruptors*. National Institute of Environmental Health Sciences. https://www.niehs.nih.gov/health/topics/agents/endocrine

84. National Institutes of Health. (2022). *Magnesium*. National Institutes of Health. https://ods.od.nih.gov/factsheets/Magnesium-HealthProfessional/

85. NHS inform. (2023, January 20). *Loss of libido*. NHS Inform. https://www.nhsinform.scot/illnesses-and-conditions/sexual-and-reproductive/loss-of-libido/

86. O'Neal, C. (2017). *Herbal and Nutritional Therapeutics for Autoimmune Hypothyroidism*. https://img1.wsimg.com/blobby/go/4816464f-c3c3-42f5-9b59-7c94a7702fdf/downloads/b48da1f1-3e2b-422b-b898-4b6f228ac654/Herbal%20Treatments%20for%20Autoimmune%20Thyroid%20Healt.pdf?ver=1734898646905

87. Oliveira, N. (2025, February 26). *Water*. The Nutrition Source. https://nutritionsource.hsph.harvard.edu/water/

88. Panossian, A., & Wikman, G. (2010). Effects of Adaptogens on the Central Nervous System and the Molecular Mechanisms Associated with Their Stress—Protective Activity. *Pharmaceuticals*, *3*(1), 188–224. https://doi.org/10.3390/ph3010188

89. Pantazi, A. C., Mihai, C. M., Balasa, A. L., Chisnoiu, T., Lupu, A., Frecus, C. E., Mihai, L., Ungureanu, A., Kassim, A., Andrusca, A., Nicolae, M., Cuzic, V., Lupu, V. V., & Cambrea, S. C. (2023). Relationship between Gut Microbiota and Allergies in Children: A Literature Review. *Nutrients*, *15*(11), 2529. https://doi.org/10.3390/nu15112529

90. Pappas, A. (2009). The relationship of diet and acne. *Dermato-Endocrinology*, *1*(5), 262–267. https://doi.org/10.4161/derm.1.5.10192

91. Piedmont. (n.d.). *Keeping your lymphatic system healthy*. Www.piedmont.org. Retrieved August 22, 2025, from https://www.piedmont.org/living-real-change/keeping-your-lymphatic-system-healthy

92. Pobiner, B. (2013). *Evidence for Meat-Eating by Early Humans*. Nature.com. https://www.nature.com/scitable/knowledge/library/evidence-for-meat-eating-by-early-humans-103874273/

93. Pollan, M. (2008). *In Defense of Food: An Eater's Manifesto* (p. 1). Penguin Press.

94. Popham, S. (2025, May 14). *The Seasonal Allergy Strategy Part 1*. The School of Evolutionary Herbalism. https://www.evolutionaryherbalism.com/2025/05/14/the-seasonal-allergy-strategy-part-1/

95. Purves, D. (2001). The Enteric Nervous System. In G. J. Augustine, D. Fitzpatrick , L. C. Katz, A.-S. LaMantia, L. McNamara, & S. M. Williams (Eds.),

Neuroscience. 2nd edition. Sinauer Associates. https://www.ncbi.nlm.nih.gov/books/NBK11097/

96. Rádis-Baptista, G. (2023). Do Synthetic Fragrances in Personal Care and Household Products Impact Indoor Air Quality and Pose Health Risks? *Journal of Xenobiotics*, *13*(1), 121–131. https://doi.org/10.3390/jox13010010

97. Riccardi, G., & Rivellese, A. A. (1991). Effects of dietary fiber and carbohydrate on glucose and lipoprotein metabolism in diabetic patients. *Diabetes Care*, *14*(12), 1115–1125. https://doi.org/10.2337/diacare.14.12.1115

98. Ross, A. E., Doxey, A. C., & Neufeld, J. D. (2017). The Skin Microbiome of Cohabiting Couples. *MSystems*, *2*(4), e00043-17. https://doi.org/10.1128/msystems.00043-17

99. Sadowsky, R. L., Sulejmani, P., & Lio, P. A. (2023). Atopic Dermatitis: Beyond the Skin and Into the Gut. *Journal of Clinical Medicine*, 12(17), 5534. https://doi.org/10.3390/jcm12175534

100. Samadi, S., Khadivzadeh, T., Emami, A., Moosavi, N. S., Tafaghodi, M., & Behnam, H. R. (2010). The effect of Hypericum perforatum on the wound healing and scar of cesarean. *Journal of Alternative and Complementary Medicine*, *16*(1), 113–117. https://doi.org/10.1089/acm.2009.0317

101. Shafik, A. (1993). Effect of different types of textile fabric on spermatogenesis: an experimental study. *Urological Research*, *21*(5), 367–370. https://doi.org/10.1007/bf00296839

102. Shah, M. G., & Maibach, H. I. (2001). Estrogen and skin. An overview. *American Journal of Clinical Dermatology*, *2*(3), 143–150. https://doi.org/10.2165/00128071-200102030-00003

103. Shankar, A. H., & Prasad, A. S. (1998). Zinc and immune function: the biological basis of altered resistance to infection. *The American Journal of Clinical Nutrition*, *68*(2), 447–463. https://doi.org/10.1093/ajcn/68.2.447s

104. Spiller, M. (2024, December 4). *Dopamine Rush - 27 Things to Do Instead of Scroll.* Sanford Behavioral Health. https://sanfordbehavioralhealth.com/2024/12/04/dopamine-rush-27-things-to-do-instead-of-scroll/

105. Srivastava, S. B. (2021). Vitamin D: Do We Need More Than Sunshine? *American Journal of Lifestyle Medicine*, *15*(4), 155982762110056. https://doi.org/10.1177/15598276211005689

106. Swift, K. (2017, November 13). *Ground Ivy: Herb of the Week.* CommonWealth Holistic Herbalism. https://commonwealthherbs.com/ground-ivy-herb-week/

107. Tassell, M. C., Kingston, R., Gilroy, D., Lehane, M., & Furey, A. (2010). Hawthorn (Crataegus spp.) in the treatment of cardiovascular disease. *Pharmacognosy Reviews,* 4(7), 32–41. https://doi.org/10.4103/0973-7847.65324

108. Taylor, K. (2020, December 10). *How Birth Control Messes Up Mutual Attraction.* Natural Womanhood. https://naturalwomanhood.org/how-the-birth-control-pill-messes-up-mutual-attraction/

109. The Health Sciences Academy. (2021). *Dangers of dehydration* [online course]. In Skincare and Repair Nutrition. https://thehealthsciencesacademy.org/advanced-skincare-and-repair-nutrition-specialist-level-5-diploma/

110. The Institute for Functional Medicine. (2025, April 22). *Nutrition and Impacts on Hormone Signaling.* The Institute for Functional Medicine. https://www.ifm.org/articles/nutrition-impacts-hormone-signaling

111. The Nutrition Source. (2018, August 6). *Straight Talk About Soy.* The Nutrition Source. https://nutritionsource.hsph.harvard.edu/soy/

112. Thompson, H. (2012, December 28). *An Evolutionary Whodunit: How Did Humans Develop Lactose Tolerance?* Npr.org. https://www.npr.org/sections/thesalt/2012/12/27/168144785/an-evolutionary-whodunit-how-did-humans-develop-lactose-tolerance

113. Tin, A. (2024, September 25). *Federal court rules against EPA in lawsuit over fluoride in water* (A. E. Gualtieri, Ed.). CBS News. https://www.cbsnews.com/news/epa-fluoride-drinking-water-federal-court-ruling/

114. U.S. Environmental Protection Agency. (2024, December 19). *Overview of Endocrine Disruption.* Www.epa.gov. https://www.epa.gov/endocrine-disruption/overview-endocrine-disruption

115. UnityPoint Health. (n.d.). *How Your Lymphatic System Works.* UnityPoint Health. Retrieved July 31, 2025, from https://www.unitypoint.org/news-and-articles/how-your-lymphatic-system-works

116. USDA National Agricultural Statistics Service. (2024). *2023 Agricultural Chemical Use Survey Soybeans.* https://www.nass.usda.gov/Surveys/Guide_to_NASS_Surveys/Chemical_Use/2023_Barley_Oats_Peanuts_Soybeans/ChemHighlights-Soybeans-2023.pdf

117. Veit, H. Z. (2018). American Food, Cooking, and Nutrition, 1900–1945. *Oxford Research Encyclopedia of American History.* https://doi.org/10.1093/acrefore/9780199329175.013.339

118. Wang, F.-Y., & Chi, C.-C. (2021). Rosacea, Germs, and Bowels: A Review on Gastrointestinal Comorbidities and Gut–Skin Axis of Rosacea. *Advances in Therapy*, *38*(3), 1415–1424. https://doi.org/10.1007/s12325-021-01624-x

119. Warren, C. M., Agrawal, A., Gandhi, D., & Gupta, R. S. (2022). The US population-level burden of cow's milk allergy. *World Allergy Organization Journal*, *15*(4), 100644. https://doi.org/10.1016/j.waojou.2022.100644

120. Weaver, J. (2021, July 12). *A fermented-food diet increases microbiome diversity and lowers inflammation, Stanford study finds.* Stanford Medicine. https://med.stanford.edu/news/all-news/2021/07/fermented-food-diet-increases-microbiome-diversity-lowers-inflammation

121. Weiss, C. (2021, November 15). *Mayo Clinic Q and A: Talking to young children about anatomy and sex.* Mayo Clinic News Network. https://newsnetwork.mayoclinic.org/discussion/mayo-clinic-q-and-a-talking-to-young-children-about-anatomy-and-sex/

122. West Bengal Chemical Industries Limited. (2025, May 16). *Hidden Link: How Mineral Deficiency Disrupts Women's Hormones.* West Bengal Chemical Industries Limited. https://www.wbcil.com/blog/the-silent-struggle-how-mineral-deficiency-is-affecting-womens-hormonal-health/

123. Wiertsema, S. P., van Bergenhenegouwen, J., Garssen, J., & Knippels, L. M. J. (2021). The Interplay between the Gut Microbiome and the Immune System in the Context of Infectious Diseases throughout Life and the Role of Nutrition in Optimizing Treatment Strategies. *Nutrients*, *13*(3), 886. https://doi.org/10.3390/nu13030886

124. Wolkodoff, N. E. (2024). Pine Pollen Impacts Testosterone-Related Symptoms in Older Men: A Pilot Report. *Annals of Clinical and Medical Case Report*, *14*(5), 1–9. https://acmcasereport.org/wp-content/uploads/2024/09/ACMCR-v14-2275-1.pdf

125. Xu, G., Liu, B., Yang, W., Snetselaar, L. G., Chen, M., Bao, W., & Strathearn, L. (2022). Association of Food Allergy, Respiratory Allergy, and Skin Allergy with Attention Deficit/Hyperactivity Disorder among Children. *Nutrients*, *14*(3), 474. https://doi.org/10.3390/nu14030474

126. Xu, G., Snetselaar, L. G., Jing, J., Liu, B., Strathearn, L., & Bao, W. (2018). Association of Food Allergy and Other Allergic Conditions With Autism Spectrum Disorder in Children. *JAMA Network Open*, *1*(2), e180279. https://doi.org/10.1001/jamanetworkopen.2018.0279

127. Yousef, H., Alhajj, M., Fakoya, A. O., & Sharma, S. (2024, June 8). *Anatomy, Skin (Integument), Epidermis.* PubMed; StatPearls Publishing. https://www.ncbi.nlm.nih.gov/books/NBK470464/

128. Zhai, Z., Liu, Y., Wu, L., Senchina, D. S., Wurtele, E. S., Murphy, P. A., Kohut, M. L., & Cunnick, J. E. (2007). Enhancement of Innate and Adaptive Immune Functions by Multiple Echinacea Species. *Journal of Medicinal Food, 10*(3), 423–434. https://doi.org/10.1089/jmf.2006.257

Indispensable Reading: (Must-Haves for Your Bookshelf)

Herbal Contraindications and Drug Interactions by Francis Brinker

Natural Remedies for Low Testosterone by Stephen Harrod Buhner

The Natural Testosterone Plan by Stephen Harrod Buhner

Wheat Belly by

William Davis, MD

The Modern Herbal Dispensatory by Thomas Easley and Steven Horne

Aphrodisiac: The Herbal Path to Healthy Sexual Fulfillment and Vital Living by Kimberly Gallagher

Finally Focused by James Greenblatt, MD and Bill Gottlieb, CHC

This is Your Brain on Birth Control: How the Pill Changes Everything by Sarah E. Hill, PhD

Healing Mushrooms by Tero Isokauppila

The Herb Book by John Lust

Energetic Herbalism by Kat Maier

Herbal Hormone Handbook for Women by Carmen Reeves

Hormone Intelligence by Aviva Romm

Taking Charge of Your Fertility by Toni Weschler

Adaptogens by David Winston

The Great Cholesterol Myth, Revised and Expanded by Jonny Bowden, PhD and Stephen Sinatra MD

Healing Lyme by Stephen Herrod Buhner

Amelia South Resources

Email Address:
amelia@nobsherbalist.com

No-BS Herbalist (website)

Social
Media

One-on-One
Consultation

Leaky Gut Quiz

Gut Healing Protocol

Wildcrafted Eats Course

Complete Stop Smoking System

End Your Emotional Eating and Sugar Addiction System

Forage and Heal: Discovering Plant Identification, Black Walnuts, and Nature's Healing Power (book)

Amelia South Resources: Short-Form Videos

Corn Silk

Evening Primrose

Fire Cider Recipe

Golden Milk Recipe Tutorial

Harvest Soup Recipe

Herbal Bitters Recipe

Herbal Steams

Hypothyroid Low Energy Quick Fix Recipe

Iron Deficiency

Naturally Healing Scalp Psoriasis

Red Clover

Stinging Nettle

Stop Urinary Incontinence

Wild Lettuce

Additional Resources:
Part One

"Why Americans don't pronounce the H in herbs" (video)

"They Might Be Giants - Roy G Biv" (video)

Harvard's guide on Recommended Daily Water Intake (web article)

"Washing Diapers" (web article)

"Is This My Body? A Manual on Navigating Child Masturbation without Shame" (research paper)

Additional Resources: Part Two

7song, "Herbal First Aid" (website)

Herbal Constituents

(website)

Layne Whitley's

Website

Bryan Redfield's

Website

The Holistic Herbalism Podcast, "Herbs for First Aid and Disaster Response" (podcast episode)

"The Ins and Outs of Holistic Nutrition for Pancreatic Health"

(web article)

"6 Ways to Do Intermittent Fasting" (web article)

Mountain Rose Herbs (website)

Nick Ortner EFT

(video)

Brad Yates EFT

(video)

"Herbal and Nutritional Therapeutics for Autoimmune Hypothyroidism" (paper)

QR Code Compatible on Some Devices –
Google "American Herbalists Guild Hypothyroid"

Recommended Products

Chapter Three:

Silver Fern™

Ultimate Probiotic

Chapter Seven:

Hema-Plex

Iron Tablets

Chapter Eight:

Silver Fern™

Postbiotic+

Chapter Ten:

Seltzer

Maker

Chapter Fifteen:

The Earthling Co.
Dry Shampoo

Re-Mineralizing
Tooth Powder

Massaging
Gum Picks

Biodegradable
Dental Floss

Water Dental
Flosser

Crystal Mineral
Deodorant

Chapter Sixteen:

Barefoot Shoes for Babies

Barefoot Shoes for Adults

Chapter Twenty:

Turmeric Supplement
with Black Pepper

Chapter Twenty-Three:

Ear Oil for Earaches
and Ear infections

Chapter Twenty-Four:

Allergy Sinus Tincture

Chapter Twenty-Five:

Lovebug Baby
Probiotic Drops

Psoriasis-Specific
Shampoo and Conditioner

Wildcrafted Witch Hazel Extract

Gua Sha Tool

Argan Oil

Carrot Seed Oil

Frankincense Oil

Rosehip Seed Oil

Sea Buckthorn Seed Oil

Aging Face Oil Blend

Bee Pollen

Powdered Collagen

Badger Mineral Sunscreen

Chapter Twenty-Six:

Wool

Dryer Balls

Pure Encapsulations Trace Minerals

Chapter Twenty-Eight:

Pine Pollen Extract

Chapter Thirty-One:

UTI-Treating Supplement

Chapter Thirty-Two:

Saluz™ AFA Wild

Harvested Blue Green Algae

Chapter Thirty-Three

Liver Support Supplement

Ox Bile

Chapter Thirty-Six

Walking Pad

Kettlebell

Rebounder

Chapter Thirty-Seven

B-Complex

Supplement

Chapter Thirty-Eight

Silver Fern™ Brand's

Stress Complex

About the Author

Amelia South is a Practicing Clinical Herbalist, Professional Foraging Instructor, Gut Health Specialist, and Self-help Coach living on her micro-farm in Eastern Connecticut. Her medicine cabinet is full of herbal concoctions, she's more interested in the weeds between your flower beds, and she loves making your eyes light up when you learn something new. She gardens and hikes barefoot and eats wild food wherever she goes.

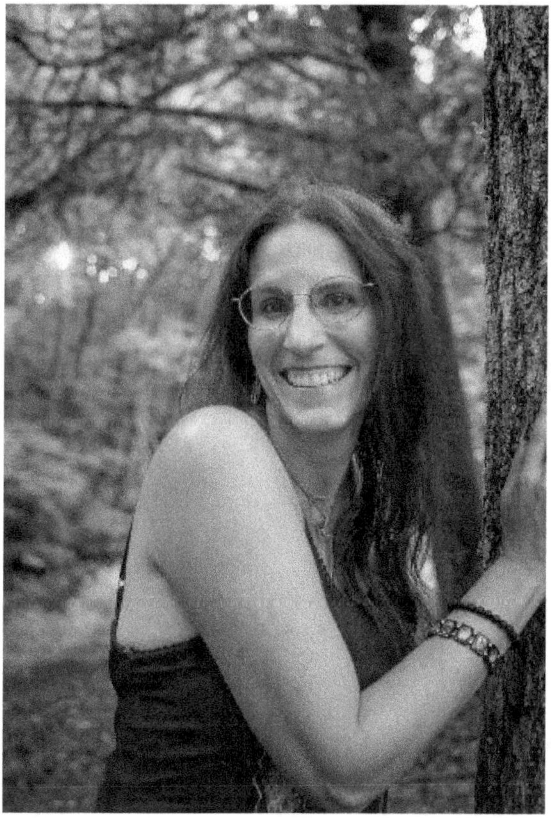

Photo by Ling Li Messer

www.ingramcontent.com/pod-product-compliance
Lightning Source LLC
LaVergne TN
LVHW052036200926
848481LV00005B/1694
* 9 7 9 8 9 9 4 4 3 2 2 0 4 *